I0100374

Two Friends

From a Life-Threatening Stroke
to a 66-Year-Old Model!

Geri Rockstein

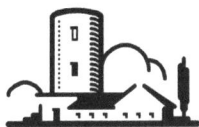

Brick Tower Press
Habent Sua Fata Libelli

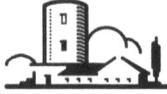

Brick Tower Press
Manhanset House
Shelter Island Hts., New York 11965-0342
Tel: 212-427-7139

bricktower@aol.com • www.BrickTowerPress.com

All rights reserved under the International and Pan-American Copyright
Conventions. No part of this publication may be reproduced, stored in a retrieval
system, or transmitted in any form or by any means, electronic, or otherwise, without
the prior written permission of the copyright holder.

The Brick Tower Press colophon is a registered trademark of
J. T. Colby & Company, Inc.

Library of Congress Cataloging-in-Publication Data
Rockstein, Geri.
Two Friends
p. cm.

1. Biography & Autobiography—Medical.
2. Health & Fitness—Diseases—Heart.
3. Health & Fitness—Diseases—Nervous System.
Nonfiction, I. Title.

ISBN: 978-1-899694-20-4, Trade Paper | ISBN: 978-1-876969-10-3, Hardcover

Cover photo by Natalia Dolan

Copyright © 2024 by Geri Rockstein

April 2024

Two Friends

*From a Life-Threatening Stroke
to a 66-Year-Old Model!*

Geri Rockstein

The publisher is not in the business of giving medical advice. If you have any questions or concerns, please consult a physician.

Dedication

This book is dedicated to helping people who've had a stroke. Or, if you have a friend or family member who's had a stroke, hopefully this book will help you too.

Table of Contents

Foreword

I met Geri at a tennis club in Montreal some 30 years ago. She had short, spiky red hair, bright red lipstick and a ferocious backhand. We quickly bonded over our shared interests including sports, fashion, family, food and wine and bargain hunting. We became the "adopted daughters" in our respective families and enjoyed spending time together. Our friendship survived a move to Toronto, me directly, Geri after a side trip to Calgary.

Suddenly life stopped. The unthinkable happened. I knew Geri had Atrial Fibrillation, but she seemed invincible to me. Yet, she had suffered a stroke. Everything changed. What would her life look like after this? I put my fears into a drawer in my brain and left it there. All that mattered now was being with Geri.

Here we are today. Geri's hair is now mainly grey and she has taken up pickleball rather than tennis. She stopped drinking after her Afib diagnosis but our other interests haven't changed. Our journey through her recovery has brought us closer together. We truly treasure our time together, but somehow that time passes much too quickly. One hour turns into two and more. I am so grateful for her friendship. She is a rock to lean on in my life, and I for her.

I love you Geri!

—Sue Foster

Introduction

An ambulance took me, unconscious, to the hospital and immediately I was given a clot-busting procedure. My best friend Sue arrived and was taken to the floor where two doctors had just finished with me and walked out of the room. The older doctor, Dr. Daniel Selchen, sat down with Sue. He told her that I had a very severe stroke and he asked what I did for a living. Sue told him - communications. He took her hand and said that life was going to be very hard and frustrating for me.

This is my story, that love, friends and family give you hope and inspiration to win back your life!

Chapter 1 – I Had a Stroke

I was lying on the floor in my bedroom wrapped in a bath towel saying to myself, "Don't close your eyes until you see someone, don't close your eyes until you see someone." I had to stay awake! On September 12, 2018 I had a stroke. I was 64 years old.

I should have been dead, but there was an angel looking out for me! And that angel was my mother, who in her heart knew that she had to live long enough to save my life. When my father Joe died six years ago, my mother Shirley told me that she wanted to die to be with Joe, but she had to stay alive for me. I was grateful that she found anything to live for. Without Shirley I would have been dead!

After Joe's death I moved Shirley into my apartment building. That way we could both be independent, but close by. Shirley and I were both very early risers. The latest we got up was 6:00am. Every morning I would go up to Shirley's apartment at 7:00am, say good morning, find out if she needed anything and tell her that I'd see her for dinner. Shirley was a gourmet cook and every night she would make a wonderful meal! I set off walking to work because I walked 10 kms/day. One morning I didn't show up at 7:00am. It was 7:15am and Shirley knew that something was wrong. She was afraid to come down to my apartment, so she called my friend Erik, who lived in the building and had my key. He walked into my bedroom. As soon as I saw Erik, I lost consciousness. I don't remember the ambulance ride or any treatment in the hospital. I just remember waking for a few minutes at a time to see my best friend Sue. I didn't know that I was in hospital. I didn't know that I was in the ICU.

For the next few days I have no memory, but my best friend Sue does.

Sue

"Geraldine has had a stroke. She's in St. Mike's." That was what I remember from my conversation with Geri's mom Shirley. I don't remember getting into the taxi, but I found myself at St. Mike's with a very nice volunteer. He found the floor where Geri was, and as good luck had it, the two doctors who had just performed a clot-busting procedure on her came out of one of the doors. I sat down with the shorter, older doctor, Dr. Daniel Selchen. He had a kind face. He told me that it was a really bad stroke and that Geri had a 1 in 4 chance of a full recovery. He asked me what she did. I said communications. He put his hand on mine and said that it will be very hard and frustrating for her. I went into the room to see Geri. She was lying on the operating table and her eyes were open. I knew she was present and that she knew who I was. I told her that Shirley was going to be okay. Then I left the room so they could move her to the ICU ward.

I decided that I would not tell Geri or anyone else about her prognosis. If anyone could beat the odds, it was Geri. So, I mentally filed it away and concentrated on the present.

I sat at Geri's bedside and held her hand. This was unusual for Geri; she didn't request handholding normally. But she reached out for my hand. I watched all the numbers of the monitors without really understanding what they meant. Her eyes were closed most of the time, but I was sure she felt my presence. I also knew that they woke her up every hour and asked her questions. I don't think she was remotely aware of this, but they did it to monitor her. By 10:00pm the nurse told me to go home and I did. As I was not a family member, power of attorney was granted to Shirley. I persuaded the staff to agree to call me if there was an issue and that I would go and be with Shirley if any decisions had to be made. The thought of her 87-year-old mother getting a call from ICU at 3:00am was terrifying.

Katherine

"A quick phone call, one question? Do you know a writer for my blogs and website?" "Of course, I know Geri Rockstein. Call her now." I made that phone call to Geri over 20 years ago. It was the beginning

not only of a professional relationship, but it quickly blossomed into a lifelong friendship not only with Geri but with her parents, Shirley and Joe, and meeting Geri's best friend Sue and her niece Erica. I have always been amazed how one phone call could lead us to a lifetime of love and friendship.

It was very early on a September morning that I received a phone call from Shirley, Geri's mother. "Katherine, Oh Katherine!" I knew something was terribly wrong. I asked Shirley what had happened. "It's Geraldine." she sobbed. "She had been rushed to the hospital. It's serious." I remember the fear and numbness that came over me. I learned later that morning Geri had experienced a stroke and was in St Michael's hospital. I was able to visit with her the next day. I arrived at the hospital. Geri's best friend and rock, Sue, was sitting on a chair next to Geri. I was relieved that Geri was at St. Michael's Hospital and undergoing excellent medical care. Even though in intensive care Geri had a smile on her face that told me she would be okay. Even though she couldn't speak, I would joke with her that she would be speaking in no time.

Judy S.

I got a call from Sue Foster to tell me about Geri's stroke. She gave me some preliminary information. I immediately asked about Shirley and asked if I could call her. I did and checked in with her a few times after that. I offered to come to Toronto to help in any way I could, but both Sue and Shirley said that there was really nothing I could do, and that Geri was being well cared for. Shirley was being covered by Geri's wonderful friends. I would really be redundant at that point. Sue told me she'd add me to the WhatsApp group, so I'd have news as it happened. It was a Godsend!

Janice

When I received the call from Sue, I said, "Hi Sue" in a cheery voice. But then I thought, wait, why is Sue calling me? It's not that I wouldn't like to hear from her, but we always met when Geri was with us. Then I asked Sue, "OH NO, is Shirley okay?" I thought perhaps Geri was too upset to call me herself. Sue replied, "No Janice, Geri would call you if that were the case." Then she told me that Geri had suffered a major stroke. I was in shock as Geri and I had just had our regular girls get together the Sunday before (she had her stoke the following Wednesday). Needless to say, I was very shocked, scared and saddened.

I called Shirley right away to see how she was doing and continued to call Shirley every few days just to talk. There was a lot she was trying to figure out with everyone and I just wanted to be there for her even though I could not do anything as I live 2.5 hrs away.

Sue

I was also in shock. I have no memory of calling Judy S. or Janice, and I don't recall who else I spoke to. I know I must have called Shirley at least twice a day to keep her up to speed with Geri's progress. Geri didn't want her mom to come to the hospital and see her while she was still in the early recovery stages. It would have been frightening to see her daughter in that state.

Geri

A few days later I became slowly aware of my reality. I had vague recollections of lying in a bed and seeing nurses walking around. I tried to talk to them, but no words came out. I had no idea that I was in ICU for a few days. Now I was in a room in a hospital and I had no idea what I was doing there! What hospital was I in? What kind of ward was it? I was in a bed, closest to the door. On my right was a curtain which I assumed blocked off the view to another patient. I didn't know what was wrong with me, or where I was!

As I looked around the room I saw Sue. She looked very happy that I opened my eyes. I tried to talk to her, but I couldn't say anything! Sue told me that I had a stroke and that I was at St. Michael's Hospital. I don't think that I really understood! How could I have a stroke? It really took a while for it to settle in. I was lying on my back and wanted to shift, but I couldn't use my right arm or hand. It would take me a while from just waking up to realizing that I couldn't talk and my arm and hand were paralyzed. I hadn't even discovered that my right leg was also paralyzed!

Nurses would come in and ask me questions and I couldn't answer them, but I understood everything. I had aphasia. Aphasia is a condition that robs you of the ability to communicate. It can affect your ability to speak, write and understand language, both verbal and written and it typically occurs suddenly after a stroke or a head injury. It certainly robbed me of my ability to speak! I was being fed by a tube because half of my face was paralyzed and they were afraid that I would choke on food. Finally, after a few days three words came back to me. I had three words in my entire vocabulary - Yes, No and Fuck! which for me was a curse because I'm a talker with a large vocabulary! In my mind I could have a whole conversation, but I couldn't say the words. They were stuck in my throat!

When I was finally coherent, Sue and I talked (Sue talked and I answered Yes or No, but Sue always understood what I wanted) about documenting my journey. I was delighted that Sue would take this on. Together we would see where it went.

Sonya

I had tried to get in touch with Geri for a couple of days. It was very unusual for her not to respond to my messages. Could she be upset with me, I thought for a brief moment. And then, I began to worry. Later that day Sue confirmed my worst fear that something terrible had befallen her.

I remember going to see Geri at St Mike's Hospital for the first time. It was a week after her stroke. I didn't know what to expect. She greeted me with hello, sitting up in her hospital bed. Geri couldn't talk except for very few words, as well, she couldn't move her right hand and arm. It didn't take long though to discover that her personality was still intact. And it's that personality that would make a huge difference in her recovery. I never witnessed her feeling sorry for herself or asking "why me?" She immersed herself in her recovery and WORKED HARD at it. Her positive attitude and strong will to get better no doubt played a significant role in her successful stroke recovery.

Pam

I didn't get to see Geri for about one week after her stroke. I had been on vacation with my mom and went to see her immediately upon my return. I knew she had suffered a stroke and thought I knew what to expect but walking into that room and seeing her in a hospital bed was just devastating. No one is prepared to see someone they care for in that situation. Geri is one of the most vibrant people I know, always moving, always busy and, if not, she'll find something to do. To see her lying there was such a shock. I knew she was still in very critical condition and she was still in grave danger. What gave me hope though was the look in her eyes. Geri was still there, all of her. It was then that I knew while she had a long road ahead, she would make it and if anyone had the capacity to fight back to a normal life, it was her. I went into that room thinking it could be good-bye and left knowing she wasn't going anywhere.

Geri

I had a roommate, but I never heard her utter a word. And I never saw her, but I saw her husband coming and going. I could not get out of bed, even to go to the bathroom because my heart and blood pressure were very unstable. I really didn't know how severe my stroke was and that getting out of bed could kill me. I was wearing diapers and I had to urinate and defecate in them. It was totally disgusting! Even when I knew that I had to go to the bathroom – it was the diapers! You have no idea how this drove me insane! I'm crazy clean. But there was one thing that gave me great peace and happiness. Each morning when I woke up, I could see my father sitting in the chair beside me, smiling wondrously, but he never said a word! He was wearing his green coat, plaid shirt and jeans. Many months later I finally realized that was why I never had a bad day or a sad day after I had my stroke. I never woke up and said, "Why me? It's not fair!" I had my father with me and he was the happiest person that I ever knew and he loved me like no other! I should have known that someone who loved me as much as he did would have never left

10

me alone. We were in this together! He would never have been sad. Joe would have just woken up, smiled and thanked God for making another day. Even when he was dying in the hospital, he was always in a great mood telling jokes. The nurses and doctors loved him and anyone that needing cheering up came to see Joe. My father gave me a piece of his attitude for living! I will be forever in his debt. And every morning when I wake up, I thank God for making another day.

Unfortunately, my mother got taken to the hospital. This was going to be a long visit! Shirley hadn't been well for about one year. She had trouble walking and was now with a walker. Something in her body was causing Shirley to blow up, and it wasn't from eating. Shirley had a lovely figure. She was 5 foot 4 inches and weighed 128 pounds. Now, I have no idea what she weighed. I was worried about Shirley!

I was so lucky that I was at St. Mike's – what everyone calls St. Michael's Hospital. It's referred to as the stroke capital of Canada and I was SO lucky that I was taken there! And the location is ideal – downtown/financial district - so anyone can come and visit using public transit or by car. My friends led by Sue, came to see me regularly and they called Shirley in the hospital and went to visit her. My friends were ABSOLUTELY FANTASTIC! Sue's boss let her bring her computer to the hospital and work beside me. I was so surprised that Josie and Rachel, whom I only worked with for six months at Scotiabank, came to see me weekly. My old friends Pam, Katherine and Everton, Sonya, Erik and Veronika were always there for me. Marla (my friend Judy S.'s daughter and I refer to her as my niece) came to see me and so did Sam, Nicole, Lisa, Richard and Daniel and Abbie! And two people that I had been friends with for over 20 years – close friends - never come to see me and never called once. It's something that I didn't understand, and still don't. How can you be CLOSE friends with someone for over 20 years and then you hear that they've had a stroke (or any other disaster) and you disappear! What did you think that I was going to want from you? Certainly, we couldn't go out to dinner or the theatre, but was that all there was? But, I've taken them all out of my address book! It's funny how some friends are amazing and it shocks you how wonderful they are! Others shock you with how miserable and selfish they are. Why were they friends with me to begin with??? It makes you wonder!

Sue

At this point I knew that Geri was not going to die, but not what her recovery would look like. In my heart I believed that she would be fine, despite the prognosis. As Geri's vocabulary continued to expand in quantum leaps, the nursing staff told me it was a sign of an excellent recovery. This also gave me great hope.

One of the more aggravating tasks was responding to a paper which had drawings of common items on it and asking Geri what they were. She was also asked what day and time it was. This was quite challenging without a clock or calendar nearby. The day I knew Geri's sense of humour had survived, was when one of the residents came by and asked her where she was, obviously hoping that she would respond with "hospital." Geri fixed the resident with a supremely withering glance and said "here." I burst into laughter.

As more friends wanted to know updates, I set up a "WhatsApp" group which turned out to be very useful. All the visitors posted comments and it helped organize who was coming and when they were coming. Luckily for me, my work was very supportive, and I spent many hours at Geri's bedside working on my laptop while she slept.

Geri

After about one week, my vocabulary started to add slowly to YES, No and Fuck – just words, no sentences. And I had a television on a wall mount in my room on the left-hand side, which was wonderful because I could use my left arm and hand. If the TV was on the right side I couldn't have used it because my right arm and hand were paralyzed. So, if there was a time that I had no friends visiting or I was up in the middle of the night and couldn't sleep, I could watch TV.

I was still very tired and used to nap during the day and I have no idea how many hours I slept at night. This was so unusual for me because I never slept more that five or six hours a night and I NEVER napped during the day.

Having all kinds of friends that come to visit you in the hospital has a tendency to make the nurses lazy. If they had something to ask me, they ignored me and just asked one of my friends; but it didn't work with my friends. They told them to ask Geri and they smiled at me. My friends didn't want me to be ignored.

And I was taken for all kinds of tests! Sue came with me for lots of them. You name it and I had it. The wonderful doctors - neurologists and cardiologists - finally found the right combination and dosages of drugs to keep my heart and blood pressure stable. I am eternally grateful to my doctors at St. Mike's!

Did you know that when you have a stroke that a neurologist and a cardiologist are a necessary part of your healthcare team?

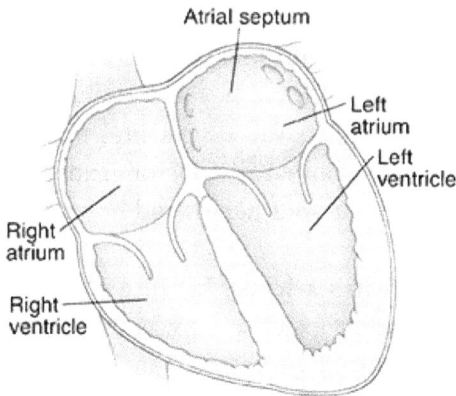

An irregular heartbeat (quiver) in the atria which could prevent all the blood flowing down to the ventricles—could create blood clots.

Neurologists and cardiologists are doctors that have a lot of specialized training in their areas. Neurologists are doctors who specialize in the brain and nervous system. This includes the spinal cord and nerves throughout the body. Because a stroke causes injury to the brain, neurologists work with people who have had strokes. Neurologists can do brain testing, manage symptoms, and recommend treatments to reduce the risk of a future stroke. Your neurologist might take scans, or pictures, of your brain to see where there is damage. And a neurologist might also test things such as your coordination, sensation, vision and reflexes. This helps to determine how your brain is working. Dr. Selchen, who Sue met after I was admitted to the hospital and was one of the doctors who did my clot-buster, is a neurologist. Before I had my stroke I had no idea that a neurologist was part of the healthcare team.

Cardiologists are doctors who specialize in the heart and cardiac system. This includes all the veins, arteries and blood vessels that carry blood around the body. Because a stroke involves the blood flow to the brain, a cardiologist is involved in your healthcare team. If you meet with a cardiologist, they will likely start with a physical examination. The doctor might order additional testing like blood work, an X-ray, or more advanced testing to look at your heart's function. I never met my cardiologist or if I did, it was at the beginning of my hospitalization and I would have no memory of it.

Neurologists and cardiologists can do testing, manage symptoms and perform procedures that your family doctor cannot do. With their help, you can learn more about your health and how to stay as healthy as possible in the future.

If you're wondering if I had a stroke because I smoked, drank too much, didn't eat well, didn't exercise or was overweight, you'd be wrong. I didn't smoke; I quit 25 years ago. I hadn't had a drink in 12 years. I ate healthy food; I never ordered in. I walked 10 kms per day. I did yoga, worked out, played golf and I wasn't overweight.

Twelve years ago I was diagnosed with atrial fibrillation or AFib.

When a person has AFib, the normal beating in the upper chambers of the heart (the two atria) is irregular, and blood doesn't flow as well as it should from the atria to the lower chambers of the heart (the two ventricles). Strokes happen when blood flow to the brain is blocked by a blood clot or by fatty deposits called plaque in the blood vessel lining.

Symptoms

According to the Mayo Clinic some people with atrial fibrillation (Afib) don't notice any symptoms. Those who do have atrial fibrillation symptoms may have signs and symptoms such as:

Sensations of a fast, fluttering or pounding heartbeat (palpitations)

Chest pain

Dizziness

Fatigue

Light headedness

Reduced ability to exercise

Shortness of breath

Weakness

I did not have any symptoms of Afib. When I was at my family doctor for my annual check up, she was taking my pulse and immediately thought that I had Afib so she sent me for a cardiogram and yes, I did have Afib.

These are the main types of atrial fibrillation:

Occasional (paroxysmal atrial fibrillation). Afib symptoms come and go, usually lasting for a few minutes to hours. Sometimes symptoms occur for as long as a week and episodes can happen repeatedly. Symptoms might go away on their own. Some people with occasional Afib need treatment.

Persistent. With this type of atrial fibrillation, the heart rhythm doesn't go back to normal on its own. If a person has Afib symptoms, cardioversion or treatment with medications may be used to restore and maintain a normal heart rhythm.

Long-standing persistent. This type of atrial fibrillation is continuous and lasts longer than 12 months.

Permanent. In this type of atrial fibrillation, the irregular heart rhythm can't be restored. Medications are needed to control the heart rate and to prevent blood clots.

My Afib started off in brief episodes and in the last year before I had my stroke, it was permanent. AFib increases a person's risk for stroke. In fact, people with AFib are five times more likely to suffer stroke. According to the Centers for Disease Control, 15 to 20 percent of ischemic strokes, which happen when blood flowing to your brain is blocked by a clot or fatty deposit, are caused by AFib. And strokes caused by complications from AFib tend to be more severe than strokes with other underlying causes.

Atrial Fibrillation and Stroke Facts According to StopAfib.org

Each year, about 795,000 people have a stroke in the U.S. About 610,000 are first attacks.

Someone has a stroke in the US about every 40 seconds.

People with nonvalvular Afib are five times more likely than someone without the condition to have a stroke; those with valvular afib have a risk 17 times higher.

An estimated 22 percent of strokes are related to Afib, a figure that has been increasing in recent years.

People with Afib are more likely to die from a stroke or be severely disabled than those without Afib.

The incidence of Afib increases with age.

Women with Afib have a higher risk of death from stroke than men.

How common is atrial fibrillation?

Some researchers have called Afib the "new cardiovascular disease epidemic of the 21st century." Afib is especially common among older adults. Over 33 million people age 55+ have been diagnosed globally. Estimates predict that 12 million people in the U.S. will have Afib by 2030. Afib causes nearly half a million yearly hospitalizations in the U.S. and leads to more and more deaths with each passing year.

After my family doctor thought I had Afib, she got me an appointment with the Director of Cardiac Arrhythmias at a major Toronto hospital. He did all kinds of tests and told me to take a Baby Aspirin (81 mg) every day. I did a lot of reading on AFib and read about what I should or shouldn't do. Alcohol was a NO NO, so I never had a drink again. Every year I went back to see him and he told me to take a Baby Aspirin, including the last year before my stroke when I told him that it was permanent and the tests showed that it was. I'm a firm believer in getting second opinions for everything, but in this case this doctor was the Director of Cardiac Arrhythmias at a major Toronto hospital. I was delighted when my family doctor got me an appointment with the Director of Cardiac Arrhythmias! I incorrectly assumed that everything he told me was absolutely accurate. Boy, was I wrong! Don't be fooled by the title!

A summary in the European Heart Journal said:

*"**Aspirin and other antiplatelets have no role in stroke prevention** (III A). The combination of anticoagulation with antiplatelets increases bleeding risk and is only justified in selected patients for a short period of time; for example, in patients with an acute coronary syndrome or stent, balancing the risk of bleeding, stroke and myocardial ischaemia (IIa B/C)."*

The European guidelines have done away with aspirin for stroke prevention. *It barely made it into our current US guidelines. I don't think aspirin should be in there and I don't think it will be there in the next guidelines. The role of aspirin will fall away," said Bernard J. Gersh, MB, ChB, DPhil, Professor of Medicine at the Mayo Clinic in Rochester, Minnesota. "It's not that aspirin is less effective than the oral*

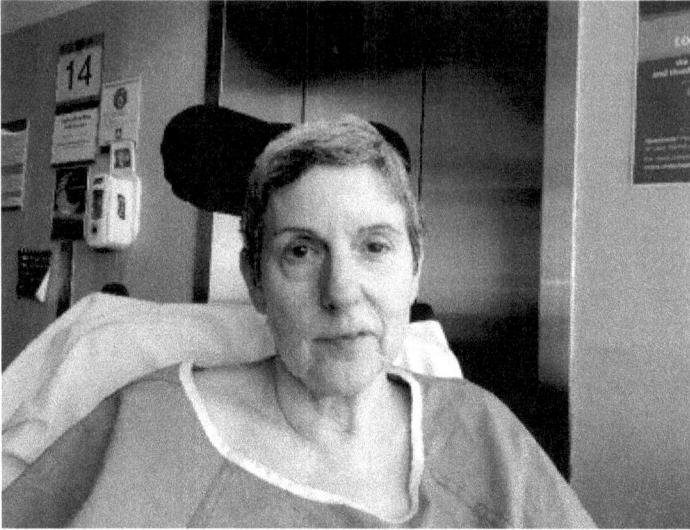

September 27, 2018
When I look at this picture of myself, it doesn't even look like me. My hair is a disaster, my face is paralyzed and were is my lipstick?????

anticoagulants, it's that there's no role for it. There are no good data to support aspirin in the prevention of stroke in atrial fibrillation."

"The use of aspirin has probably been misguided, based upon a single trial which showed a profound effect and was probably just an anomaly," said N.A. Mark Estes III, MD, Professor of Medicine and Director of the New England Cardiac Arrhythmia Center at Tufts University in Boston, and a past president of the Heart Rhythm Society.

"... I would just take it off of your clinical armamentarium because the best available data indicate that it doesn't prevent strokes. I'm certainly not using it in my patients. Increasingly in my patients with a CHA2DS2-VASc of 1, I'm discussing the risks and benefits of a novel oral anticoagulant," said Dr. Estes.

I needed a proper anticoagulant (a proper blood thinner that prevent strokes), not Baby Aspirin. So, a happy, healthy 64-year-old woman had a stroke. Needless to say, I never saw that doctor again!!! When his secretary called to tell me that it was time for my yearly checkup, I told her that I was seeing another doctor. No matter what is wrong with you, and no matter what your doctor's position is, PLEASE get a second opinion.

My doctors at St Mike's prescribed:

Dabigatran, sold under the brand name Pradaxa among others. It is an anticoagulant used to treat and prevent blood clots and to prevent stroke in people with atrial fibrillation.

Diltiazem is a calcium channel blocker. It works by relaxing the muscles of your heart and blood vessels. It is used to treat certain heart rhythm disorders.

Atorvastatin belongs to a group of medicines called **statins**. It is taken to prevent heart attacks and strokes.

Finally, I was properly medicated!!! My AFib is now occasional and definitely not severe.

Thanks to the doctors at St. Mike's I was able to be moved to a chair and use a wheelchair with someone pushing me to get out of the room. Every morning the nurses got me out of bed and into my chair. My right leg was starting to move. But, I only had one available hand (right hand and arm still paralyzed), so I could have only gone in circles! Sue was my "driver." We went down to the coffee shop on a regular basis.

After about two weeks I got another roommate. Quite honestly, I never saw the first one leave, but the new one talked a blue streak. I never saw her because she obviously was not allowed out of bed.

A week before I was moved to a rehabilitation facility called Bridgepoint, two physiotherapists came to see me twice to take me walking. It was so exciting to get up and walk – very SLOWLY and not very far. My right leg was very weak, but I was determined to get it strong again. And I was able to eat mush. Yum! Three days before I was moved to Bridgepoint I started eating solid food. Oh My God! The nurse brought me a tuna sandwich!!!! You have no idea how wonderful it felt to chew and swallow – even if it was a tuna sandwich, not my favourite. After 4.5 weeks of being cared for at St. Mike's I was going to Bridgepoint Rehab to start my work on getting my life back! I couldn't wait!

Chapter 2 – I'm in Rehab

I was released for rehab to Bridgepoint in a stretcher and taken to Bridgepoint in what looked like an ambulance, but it was a patient transfer service. Bridgepoint is a leading provider of stroke rehabilitation care, recognized with the Stroke Distinction designation from Accreditation Canada for high quality care and innovation. Stroke rehabilitation supports patients in getting back to their lives after a stroke. The care team helps patients regain function in order to enhance independence. They also help patients adapt to changes in their abilities caused by stroke. Rehabilitation is tailored to each patient's individual needs and goals.

When I arrived at Bridgepoint I was greeted with a wheelchair. They brought me to my room on a ward where there were only stroke patients. Bridgepoint is a lovely facility, but it's not as easy for people who are coming to visit. It's on Broadview Avenue, which is east of downtown, so visitors would have to take the subway and a streetcar, or drive. But I was so lucky that St. Mike's sent me to Bridgepoint! They have the best rehab in the city, which I didn't find out until much later! And the rooms were beautiful! They were very large and spacious. There were beautiful windows that allowed lots of sun to come in. I had a very large corner room with plenty of light and I had a roommate. She looked like she was in her 80s, but unfortunately she didn't speak a word of English – only Polish. Her daughter or son were there every day to translate for her. And she cried a lot! I quickly found out that at the age of 64, there was no one in my age group. They all seemed to be in their 80s and above!

Two Friends

I finally got rid of my diapers - YEAH! Of course, I had no clothes because when I was admitted to St. Mike's I was lying on the floor of my bedroom with a towel. I had to wear the hideous hospital gowns until my friend Pam (who lives in my building) brought me some clothes, sneakers and G-strings!!!! I would finally feel like a quasi-person again.

We all had TVs, but you had to pay the company for its use, so I did. Unfortunately, it never worked properly – not just mine, everyone's. Every time it didn't work, I called with a few words that I had to demand a credit. It turned out that after 4.5 weeks at Bridgepoint, I only paid $30!! Great deal, but not a lot of TV!

There was a dining room, but they never served a meal in it. Instead, when there was a lecture for patients, it was in the dining room. That was really too bad because I'm an extrovert and I would have loved to have people to talk to. Instead, we were served meals either in bed or in a chair and table beside our beds. I never went into bed until it was bedtime, so I ate beside my bed. They came around with menus and we got to choose what we wanted. It wasn't gourmet dining, but since I hadn't eaten in over a month, it was pretty good!

I had a fabulous doctor named Dr. Heather MacNeill and she had wonderful residents. She was the Director of Stroke Rehabilitation at the Sinai Health System (Bridgepoint is part of the Sinai Health System). She was my doctor at Bridgepoint and continued to see me when I was in outpatient therapy and for four months after that.

The day after I arrived, I started therapy – still in the blue hospital gowns because my clothes hadn't arrived yet. They gave me socks with sticky bottoms. Every ward had it's own workout facility. It was very large and had plenty of equipment – all new! And it had plenty of sunlight! I had one hour of speech therapy, one hour of occupational therapy and one hour of physical therapy, five days a week. I told them that wasn't enough. I had a lot of work to do and I needed all the help I could get, so they gave me an additional one hour with the assistant to the occupational therapist. On day six we had a physiotherapist who came into Bridgepoint to give us therapy. He was great and so I was busy with therapy six days a week!

What do speech therapists, occupation therapists and physical therapists do for stroke patients? Speech therapists are tasked with assessing, diagnosing, and treating speech and communication disorders. They examine language, vocal patterns, and even swallowing for a better understanding of a condition with the hopes that they will help their patients attain better communication skills. Occupational therapists work to facilitate and improve motor control and hand function in the stroke-affected upper limb and to maximize the person's ability to undertake his or her own personal self-care tasks and domestic tasks. The goal of physical therapy is to improve strength, balance, coordination, endurance and flexibility.

I started speech therapy with Ryan. He was the most amazing person – always smiling and looked like he was having fun when he probably was frustrated as hell with me! When I started with Ryan, I could say a few words but not ONE sentence. Ryan tried sneaky ways for me to say words and to make them into sentences. What ever he did was working because my vocabulary grew, but it took a while until I could make sentences. At the end of his work day, he sometimes came over to my room to see how I was doing. He was so wonderful that we are still in touch today! And Bridget, who was part of Ryan's team, treated me one day per week. She was terrific!

All of my therapists at Bridgepoint were fabulous! And I was making progress with all of them. My occupational therapist was working on my hand and my arm. The assistant occupational therapist did some wonderful things for me. Every day in addition to doing exercises with me, she also hooked my right hand up to a machine that gave electrical current for one half hour every morning. The reason that she did this was because the brain uses chemical and electrical signals to tell your muscles when to move. When a stroke occurs, the damaged parts of the brain can no longer send these signals properly. As a result, it can become difficult, if not impossible, to move your affected muscles. This is where electrical stimulation can help.

* * *

Electrical stimulation works by placing non-invasive electrodes on your skin. Once activated, these electrodes send mild electrical impulses to your muscles, causing them to contract. Electrical stimulation for stroke patients can help to activate the damaged portions of the brain by providing intense stimulation. In turn, this stimulation engages neuroplasticity, the process the brain uses to rewire itself and heal from injuries like stroke.

*   *   *

My physical therapist was working on my leg. I had my warmup on a bicycle. She wanted me to use my right hand to grip the handlebars. I couldn't do it, but I kept trying!

I was finally feeling like a quasi-person again. My wonderful friend Pam did my laundry every week and brought me clean clothes and my G-strings! Pam also brought my sneakers, which my nurse had to tie for me. As soon as I was released, I had to get sneakers that didn't have ties. I had no idea when I was going to be able to use my right hand again.

Every morning, around 7:30am, a super nurse came to take me to the bathroom in my room for a shower. I think that I was the only person that was awake, but she knew that I had been up for hours and that I loved my shower in the morning! She put me in a wheelchair and rolled me into the bathroom. There was a chair in the shower. I got out of the wheelchair and onto the chair. The nurse put on the water and gave me soap and shampoo which I did myself. Then I got up from the chair and walked over to the wall that had a bar and a towel on the floor. She dried me, dressed me and put me back in my wheelchair. Unfortunately, I couldn't wear any makeup! I never woke up and saw a day without my MAC's Russian Red lipstick, mascara and blush-on. I could have applied it because I'm ambidextrous, but half of my face was paralyzed, so no makeup for me! Then I went back to the chair and the table beside my bed. Hopefully I could watch something on TV while I was waiting for breakfast. I started my treatments at 9am. My first one everyday was with the assistant occupational therapist and I was excited!

I made such good progress with my therapists that after one week, I was finished with the wheelchair. I told them to take it out of my room because I just didn't want to look at it. I was now walking with a cane. I couldn't use a walker because I only had one hand, so I would only go in circles! After two weeks my physical therapist took me for a walk outside with a cane. We walked to Broadview, walked along the shops and back again. It was very scary! I hadn't been outside in almost two months and I really wasn't walking very well. I kept looking down on the sidewalk to make sure that I wasn't going to trip over anything. But, I did it and I couldn't wait to do it again!

Katherine

As Geri's health improved, she was off to Bridgepoint to recover, and recover she did. My husband Everton and I would visit with Geri and she would always be so pleased to show us her improvement by lifting her arm a bit. Every visit her arm went higher and her speech improved.

Sue

It was amazing to see Geri's progress; the brain is remarkable. Her vocabulary came back in leaps and bounds. Frequently, she could manage a sentence and be missing one word. It was frustrating but also very funny. We laughed and swore a great deal. Another challenge was remembering passwords for online banking. We ended up calling the credit union and with Geri's verbal permission, I was able to access her accounts and pay bills.

Geri

My credit union – Meridian – was wonderful. I never gave anyone the rights to use my account because lived alone, and I never thought anything like this would happen, but it did. Sue called them and explained about my stroke and that I really couldn't speak very well. So they asked if they could speak to me and ask me questions that would only have a Yes or No answer. It was great! With their questions and my Yes or No answers, they gave Sue access so she could pay my bills.

Thank God I was starting to make sentences again! When Sue and I were talking, and I was making a sentence, I could be missing a word. Hysterically, I used the word Jamaica for the missing word. I haven't got a clue why, except for the fact that Sue and I once had a vacation in Jamaica, but we also had a vacation in Cuba. Never-the-less I continued to use Jamaica throughout my recovery! We laughed!

I had an extraordinary nurse who taught me how to dress myself with one hand. She was the same nurse that came to take me for my shower at 7:30am. One of her best tricks was that she even showed me how to put on a bra with one hand! This is very necessary because I'm a 36D and running around without a bra is revolting! I was getting very good at doing lots of things with one hand.

I was not allowed to get out of bed without a nurse, but I started doing it anyways, and although they were not too pleased, they finally realized that I could not be stopped! I got up at 4:00am because we went to bed quite early. All I wanted to do was get out of bed and walk, so I did! Since I couldn't tie my sneakers, I just tucked the ties into my shoes.

My Polish roommate got moved to a private room because she spent a lot of time crying. Her replacement was a lovely woman who was 93. She had a daughter and sons who were with her all day and night. One of the problems on Bridgepoint's stroke floor was that I had no one to speak to who was under 80. But, I was very lucky; my friends came to visit regularly – Sue, Pam, Katherine and Everton, Judy K., Sonya, Erik, Veronika, Nicole, Abbie, Josie, Rachel, Caroline and her daughter Stella, Donald and Sam.

* * *

I was starting to improve a lot at Bridgepoint. My speech was still lousy – I couldn't make really good sentences, but I was getting better. I really tried!!!! I could now walk with a cane and started to walk without one. If I left my ward, I had to take my cane. I loved getting out and going downstairs for coffee – they had a Tim Hortons - and just sitting around on a sofa looking outside. My right leg was very weak, but getting stronger. My right arm and hand were still paralyzed.

Sue and John (Sue's husband) and Kyser (their delicious dog) came to visit. Of course John and Kyser couldn't come up, but

Sue was taking me outside for a walk to a coffee shop called the Rooster Coffee House on Broadview. It was very exciting!! I didn't have a coat, but they brought me one of John's. We walked **VERY SLOWLY** and I walked with a cane! I think the coffee shop was only about a block and a half away, but it seemed like forever! It was really something for me who was used to walking 10 kms a day. We sat outside and John and Kyser came to join us. I had a lovely latte and something from the patisserie. I could have stayed there all afternoon! We walked back to Bridgepoint and I was so proud that I made it to the coffee shop and back! Sue continued to take me to the Rooster Coffee House. I loved it!!! It was the first normal thing that I did since I was hospitalized for my stroke.

*   *   *

I was so excited that Janice came in from Kingston to visit me! We'd been **VERY** close friends

for 25 years. Every month we got together. If Shirley was well, I went to Janice's for the weekend and visited with Len and the boys – Ty and Ryker – and the animals! If Shirley wasn't well, Janice and I met in Belleville for the day. As long as we got together, it was great! Janice walked into my room and started to cry (Janice is not a crier). I guess I looked like SHIT and NO MAKEUP! Now that I look at the pictures of me at the coffee shop, I know why she cried! Sue was there and we took Janice to the Rooster Coffee House. It was a fantastic visit for me, but it must have been very difficult for Janice. I guess it must have been very difficult for all of my friends, but at the time, I really didn't get it. I woke up everyday with work to do. I didn't think of anything else.

Two Friends

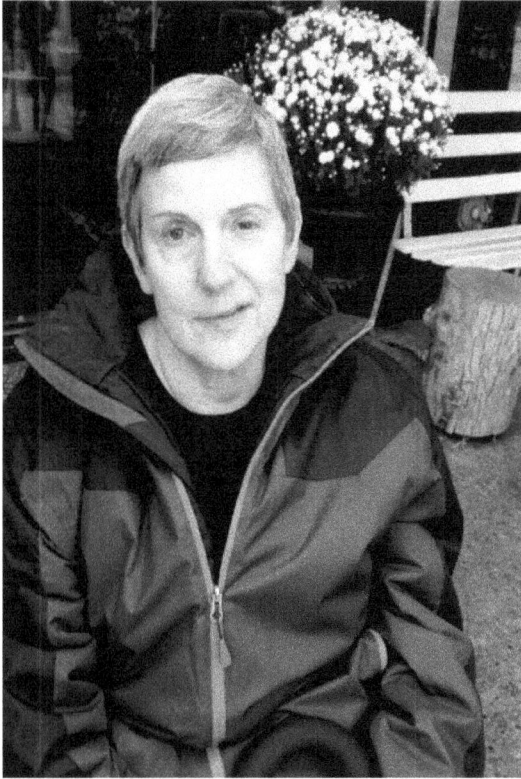

Here's a picture of me, half my face paralyzed, wearing John's jacket,
outside the Rooster Coffee House.
You can see my cane handle at the bottom center of the picture.

Janice
*I wasn't able to visit Geri until October but Sue kept us all updated
via WhatsApp. What an amazing job she did! When I did see Geri,
it was extremely hard. I told myself I was going to be very strong for
her, yet the moment I saw her I began to cry. Just the emotion I guess of
seeing someone that you love being very ill. And Geri is never short of
words so her not being able to speak was extremely hard to process. Geri*

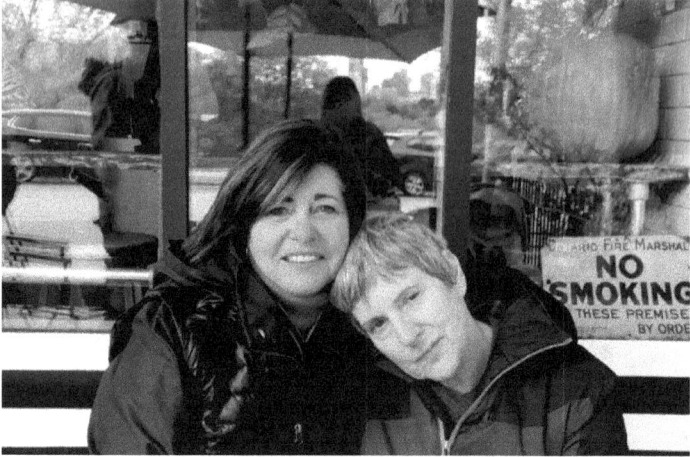

Janice & Me.

told me in the few words that she could say, "Don't cry, I'm okay."
Always a pillar of strength, she is!

We had a great visit! We met Sue and John down the street for
lunch and I was absolutely amazed at how far Geri was able to walk.
She just rested her arm on me but she walked all the way out of the
room, down the long hallway, to the elevator, down another hallway to
the front doors, then down the long entrance into Bridgepoint, and then
we continued down the block to the Rooster Coffee House. All the time,
Geri was very happy to be up and about. Then we repeated the walk
back to Bridgepoint again. Incredible!! NOTE: I was wearing a red
turtleneck just for Geri because she loves red and I always wear a
turtleneck. Haha!

Geri

I woke up every day and I had work to do. I didn't spend
much time in front of the mirror because it would have driven
me insane. Anyone that knows me can vouch for the fact that I

28

don't even throw out the trash without my MAC Russian Red lipstick, my mascara and my blush.

Katherine gave me a fabulous necklace – the second one! The first one, also fabulous, she brought to the hospital. Katherine and I have the exact same taste – we love big, gaudy jewelry! My old friends scattered around Canada and the U.S.A. called me (I had my cell phone working now) and sent presents. Marlene and Stefan from San Diego sent me a gorgeous scarf, perfume and chocolate. My old friends from BMO in Wisconsin – Teresa and Erin – sent me a red Chanel nail polish and slippers. My friend Willa from Calgary sent me two books and they were wonderful! I didn't know how to thank them!

Judy and Lenny S. even came in from Montreal to visit me! It was so wonderful! Their daughter Marla had come to see me and let Judy and Lenny know how I was doing. Judy and I have been VERY CLOSE friends for 51 years! Our fathers introduced us at the local ski hill – La Reserve - when we bought a country house in Lanthier, Quebec, close to where Judy's family had their house. Our fathers knew each other forever! Judy and I met and we were instant friends – friends forever! Judy and Lenny were better actors than Janice; they didn't cry. We went down to the coffee shop in Bridgepoint and sat on the sofas and talked (as well as I could). It was fabulous to spend the afternoon with Judy and Lenny!

Judy S.

We met on the ski hill. Besides instant friendship, there was instant competition. Geri is very focused and strives to excel in everything she does. She was always a better skier than I was. She got her buckle boots first, then her metal skis first. In spite of this, we had a wonderful adolescence of ski adventures, singing Puff the Magic Dragon and The Yodel Song on the chair lifts.

Once we were both working, we took a ski trip to Austria and Switzerland. We skied in the Alps, drank too much, avoided double black diamond hills (when we could!) and had a marvellous adventure. The Yodel Song was very prominent!

Lenny and I made the trip from Montreal to visit Geri. She was the main agenda, although our daughter, Marla, lives in Toronto as well. As we got off the elevator at Bridgepoint, I saw Geri walking in the distance. I swallowed hard and took a deep breath. She was wearing a loose, baggy top over leggings. She was walking with a cane, and her right arm was hanging limp at her side. I was prepared, but the visual was startling. We had a lovely afternoon together in the coffee shop, but it was exhausting. Geri was still having difficulty speaking, so she was working hard to express herself, and we were working hard to understand her. But we appreciated the amazing progress she was making, from no walking or talking at all, to her current level.

Sue

Compared to a hospital, Bridgepoint is a lovely spacious facility. Geri's room was large and bright. She had a TV that never worked and a nice view. I could see her spirits rising as she continued to improve. She could even wear her own clothes and one of her good friends, Pam, took care of laundry for her. At this stage, Geri was much more mobile, and we had the great treat of taking her out to the local coffee shop. She walked well with a cane. She was also able to grant me Power of Attorney and set me up to manage her financial affairs.

Geri

Bridgepoint thinks of everything for their patients! There were two lawyers who came to Bridgepoint and offered free legal services. I requested a meeting with them and they asked me what I wanted. I told them that I wanted to give Sue, Power of Attorney. They drew up the papers and Sue had Power of Attorney! It's amazing the things that you never think of when you're healthy. So **PLEASE**, be smarter than me and make sure that someone has Power of Attorney and has access to you bank account with passwords!

I was very lucky that my old friend Jane, who lives in Beamsville, is brilliant at insurance and works for Desjardins Insurance. When I was 40, we were talking about insurance. Jane knew everything and I knew nothing, but I trusted her. She created a package of Extended Health Coverage which covers things that our medical insurance doesn't – dental coverage, physiotherapy and drugs, Critical Illness covers you if you have a heart attack, stroke or cancer and Independent Living Insurance which covers you if you need help with two basic functions for living. It was a lot of money, but I bought the package. I was in perfect health, but I made the payments every month.

Thank God I had Critical Illness Insurance! I had been working on contract for 30 years, so when I had my stroke, I was not entitled to any benefits. It never mattered to me because I was never planning to retire. When people would ask me when I was planning to retire, I said, "When the morgue truck picks me up." But now I was 64 and I didn't know if I could ever work again. There certainly wasn't enough pension for me to live on at age 64. But Critical Illness paid me enough money to live on, until my full pension kicked in. I don't know what I would have done without Jane. I couldn't have paid my rent, or anything else for that matter. My Extended Health Coverage would continue until I was 65 and my Independent Living Insurance still exists. Jane made sure that if I paid it for longer than 10 years, it would exist whether I continued to pay it or not. And if I didn't use the money while I was alive, it would go to my beneficiary when I died. Thank you Jane!!!

Make sure that you speak to an expert on insurance. You'll never know when you need it, but if you do, you can't live without it! And you need to get it quite early in life because once you're on any medication, you can't get covered.

Sue
Geri asked Jane to send the cheque to my house. I remember the day it arrived. I was terrified of either losing it or being robbed. I was convinced anyone could take one look at me and know that I was trying to hide something!

Geri
THINGS THAT YOU ABSOLUTELY NEED TO DO!
   1.   Set up a Power of Attorney

2.   Make sure that someone can use your bank account and has all the passwords

3.   Invest in a Critical Illness Policy and Independent Living Insurance

4.   Display a list of medications, health conditions, your health card number

5.   Get a will

6.   Ensure that you have a support team

7.   Take good care of your health

As I was getting closer to going home, my Occupational Therapist took me to a room that had all kinds of therapy aids that I would need at home. I tried all kinds of different ones to see which ones I would like to use, so when I was released, I would go and buy them. I would need a bench for the shower and steps up to the bed.

My physical therapist taught me how to walk stairs. I was terrified!!!! But slowly and surely, I made some progress. Stairs were my worst enemy for a long time!

A week before I was finally released, Bridgepoint requested a family meeting which for me meant that Sue joined the group. Shirley, unfortunately was now in the Toronto Rehab for what was to be a very long visit. My therapists, doctor and resident and a lawyer were there. They talked about my case and what I would be able to do and not do once I got home. I was shocked because I really never heard a doctor speaking about my case before and I had no idea how severe it was. I didn't care. I was going to get back to normal again!

Sue
Right after the meeting Geri asked me if I had known how severe her stroke was. I told her about my meeting with Dr. Selchen when she had just arrived at St. Mike's and what he had said about her 1 in 4 chance of a full recovery. She had already defied the odds and greatly exceeded all expectations.

Geri

Ryan, my speech therapist, applied for me to get Wheel-Trans. Wheel-Trans is a paratransit system in Toronto, Ontario, Canada, provided by the Toronto Transit Commission. It provides specialized door-to-door accessible transit services for persons with physical disabilities using its fleet of accessible minibuses or contracted accessible taxis. And it costs virtually nothing – you pay the same fare as you would if you were riding the subway, streetcar or bus. At that time, it cost me $2.00 per ride. You can give them a transit token or pay them $2.00 in cash.

I couldn't drive because once you have a stroke they immediately notify the Ministry of Transportation and they suspend your license. I couldn't speak very well or walk very well, so Wheel-Trans would be a great option for me. And, I could go broke taking taxis, especially because Shirley was now in Toronto Rehab and I wanted to visit her every day.

Bridget, who worked with Ryan, made me cards that said "My name is Geri Rockstein. I live at 301-567 Avenue Road." This was fantastic because I was just starting to speak again and there were times that the words would not come out. It happened several times when I took a taxi home from visiting Shirley and I couldn't find the words. Thank you Bridget!

I was ready to go home!

Chapter 3 – I'm Home

After nine weeks in the hospital and in rehab, I was ACTUALLY going home. I couldn't believe it! I was excited, but also nervous. What could I do? What couldn't I do? I had so much work to do to be ME again! But, I was ready!

There was an attendant who had come to take me home in a taxi. We had to stop off at my pharmacy and get my prescriptions filled. When I walked in, my pharmacist, Andy, looked at me and told me to sit down. They made me as comfortable as possible while they very quickly filled my prescriptions. Then we went home! The attendant walked me into the building where I lived for 25 years. And there was Milan, my superintendent for the last 20 years. He gave me a big hug and a kiss and told the attendant that he was taking over and sent her home. Milan brought me up to my apartment and got me settled. My apartment was spotlessly clean because someone had called my cleaning lady, Irene, and got her back on the job. The only difference is now she's going to have to do my laundry. I have limitations with one hand.

I was joyfully home and had outpatient therapy Monday and Thursday afternoons (it started a few weeks after I was released). I couldn't cook because I could only use my left hand at first. I thought that it would be easy for me because I'm ambidextrous, but I had no idea that everything really requires two hands. Try opening a bottle of Perrier with one hand! Sue took me grocery shopping every Saturday (I bought prepared food that I could microwave) but my first day home we went out for sushi lunch. It was a great day!

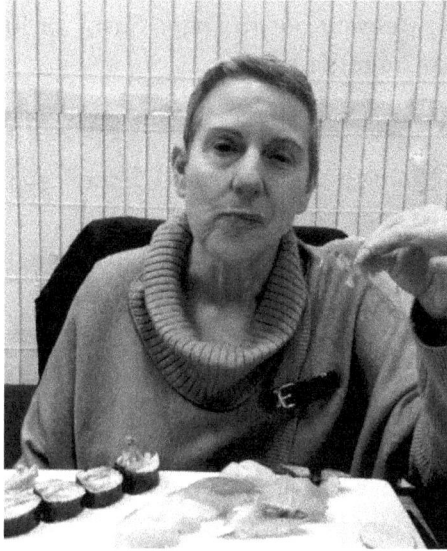

I certainly wasn't pretty, but I was happy!!

Sue

It was great that Geri was home. We live about ten minutes apart by car and thanks to my supportive husband, I was able to spend a lot of time with Geri on the weekends. We talked every day and she kept me updated on her progress. The doctor had advised that Geri would experience the most rapid recovery in the first six months, then additional recovery for up to two years.

Geri

The first day I was home Sue picked me up and took me to see my hairdresser and I got my hair cut! And then she took me to Starkmans to pick up the bench for the shower, a shower mat and the stairs to get into the bed. I used the shower bench for one month and continued to use the steps up to the bed for another month. When I was done with the bench and the steps, I gave them to Pam to bring them to her mother's seniors building. Someone could certainly use them and they weren't chea! After that we went out to Daeco Sushi for lunch. It's our absolutely favourite restaurant!

My first night at home Lisa and Richard brought me some wonderful home cooked food! Thank you Lisa and Richard!

It was the first time that I was alone in nine weeks! My friend Pam insisted that I call her every morning to let her know that I was okay. Katherine called me every morning to see that I was okay. And of course, Sue didn't miss a day. I didn't lock my front door in case I needed help. It's perfectly safe in my building to leave the door unlocked. The building is 70 years old and there has never been a robbery, so I was not nervous at all. One of the first things that I did was to order Phillips Lifeline. You wear it around your neck and if you fall, it checks in with you first and then calls the paramedics if need be. I really didn't know how I'd be at home alone. I could barely walk and I had no balance, so I really had to protect myself. The person from Phillips came over and showed me how to work it and set it up for me.

Taking a shower was a little scarier. I bought the bench and Milan set up for me, but I still had to walk into the tub. Every morning it got a little easier.

I finally sat down at the computer, but I only had one hand. I moved the mouse over to my left side and used my left hand. It was so odd – when you do something forever and then you have to change how you do it, it's very difficult! I had to type with only my left hand! I kept looking at my right hand and asking it when it was going to get back in the game!

For the last 20+ years I had a smoothie for breakfast – cashew milk, frozen mangos, a banana and lactose free yogurt, but you need two hands to make them. So, no smoothies for me! I bought croissants and had them with decaffeinated green tea in the morning. And it's amazing what you can find frozen that can go in your microwave. That's what I had for lunch and dinner. It worked out really well because I didn't have to wash many dishes. And I ate tons of fruit – bananas, apples, pears, peaches – any kind of fruit that didn't have to be peeled, except the bananas which were quite easy, even with one hand.

I walked up three stairs to get into bed. To get out I didn't need them. I couldn't make the bed which drove me nuts because I'm crazy clean and meticulous. My bedroom looked like a disaster!

You don't know how badly I wanted two hands!

Shirley was now in Toronto Rehab. We hadn't seen each other in nine weeks and I cried!!! It was wonderful!!! Shirley was not in good shape, but at least we were now together! She could never have survived coming to see me in the hospital or rehab. It would have killed her! I went every day except for Mondays and Thursdays when I had outpatient therapy. Shirley shared a room with a lovely woman who also had a daughter who came to visit. She had exercise two days a week, which is odd because at Bridgepoint you have exercise six times a week,

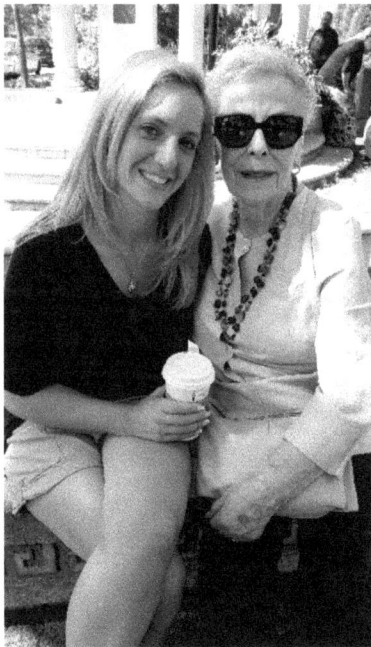

Shirley was BEAUTIFUL and looked like a model until she was 86 years old. Here is a picture of her at 85 with her granddaughter Erica (my late brother David's daughter).

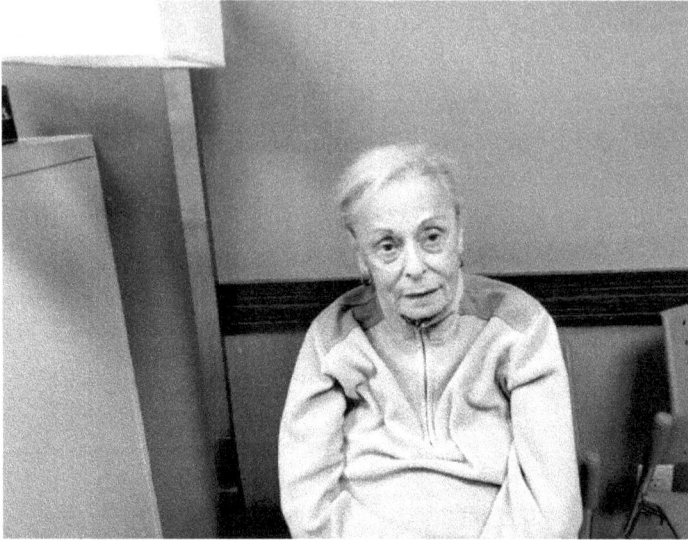

After the age of 86, Shirley's body went to hell, but her mind
was sharp as a tack!

regardless of your age. Even my 93 year old roommate had exercise six
days a week. It seems that everyone at Toronto Rehab only had exercise
two days a week! I foolishly thought that every rehabilitation facility
would give the same quality of care, but that's not so! Bridgepoint –
therapy six times per week. Toronto Rehab – therapy two times per
week. WOW!!!

Shirley's ward had a large living room with a television. I had some
issues with a few nurses on her ward or rather they had issues with me.
One of them expected me to take Shirley over to Mount Sinai Hospital
for a test with her wheelchair. Toronto Rehab and Mount Sinai Hospital
are connected by an underground tunnel. I tried to explain to her that
I just had a stroke and I didn't have the use of my right hand and arm
and couldn't walk very well either. She didn't think that was a good
enough excuse! Obviously, I didn't take her and Shirley missed her
appointment. This same, bitchy nurse continued to do the same nasty
things. She didn't believe that I didn't have the use of my right hand

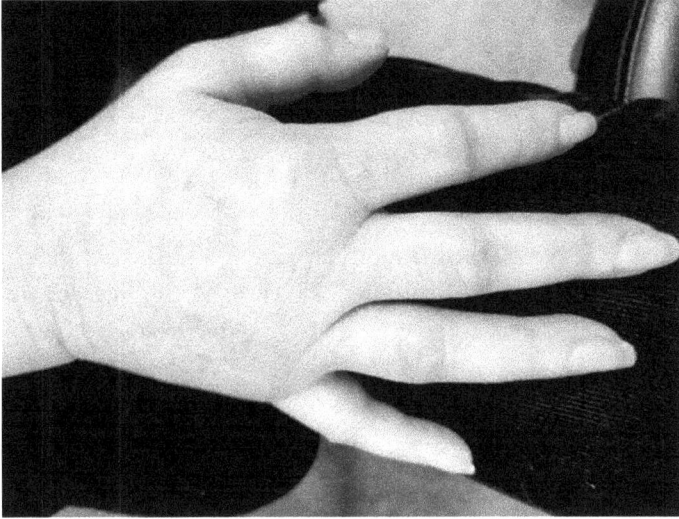

My right hand could only move a bit and it was **VERY** swollen. In fact, it looked like a giant claw!

and arm. Another nurse (who did believe me) pushed Shirley's wheelchair over to Mount Sinai for her test. I walked along with them.

Two weeks after I came home, I had an appointment to go back to St. Mike's and see Dr. Selchen, one of the doctors, the neurologist, that performed my clot-buster. I took a taxi to St. Mike's (my Wheel-Trans hadn't kicked in yet). I got called into the office and there was a very nice woman who did all kinds of tests and checked me out thoroughly. Then Dr. Selchen came in. He was just lovely! He read all the reports, smiled and said, "Angel, walk." So of course, I did. Then he said, "Angel, walk around the other way." Of course, I did. I think that he was shocked that I was walking without a cane. He had a big smile on his face and said, "I'll bet you going to have trouble with your thumb." We both started laughing and I promised him that I would call and tell him about my thumb. Six months later, I did!

Then I began outpatient therapy. By then my Wheel-Trans had kicked in. I found out pretty early that you have to give yourself at least one half hour longer that you think you need because I showed up late for my appointment. Anyone that knows me understands that I show up 10 – 15 minutes early for every appointment. You never know how many people they have to pick up and where their destinations are. But, Wheel-Trans is a GREAT service. For $2, you are picked up and for $2 you're taken home. If you have to give yourself more time, big deal!

The outpatient therapy was magic! I had the best occupational and physical therapists on the planet. On my first visit the three of us sat together and they wanted to know what I wanted from them. I told them that I wanted to be absolutely NORMAL again. I wanted to be ME! They listened and believed me. They gave me a workout program to do and so seven days a week I did an hour of physical exercise at home in the morning, even when I was coming in for therapy. And my right arm and hand started moving again - slowly! My occupational therapist told me that when I wanted to do something with my right hand that I should try and move it.

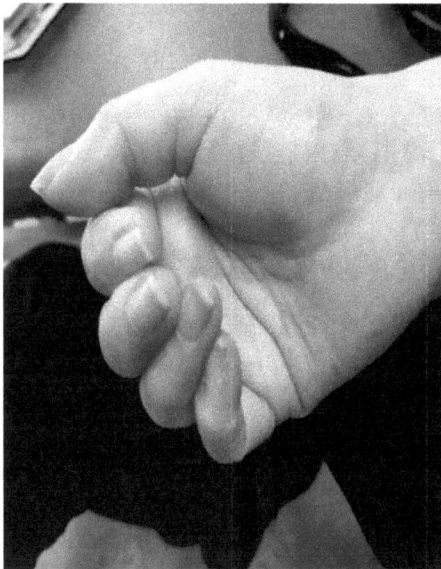

This was as much as I could move it, but I was excited because I could feel it!

I continued with my home workout every day and that really made a difference. Every day when I came into therapy, I could do more exercises or different exercises than the previous time. When I looked at the other patients that came in at the same time as I did, they just kept doing the same things that they had done before. My home workouts were really paying off. And my hand was really improving. My occupation therapist gave me a pen and paper and I started to write the alphabet! It wasn't exactly beautiful writing (I never had beautiful writing), but I wrote it.

They also made an appointment with someone who was going to counsel me on getting back to work. The woman seemed very nice until she informed me that she wanted me to do a brain scan. Dr. Heather MacNeill didn't need a brain scan, but a career counsellor did! This absolutely shocked me! I walked out of her office and reported her to the person in charge of the outpatient therapy. Even she seemed shocked. I never went back to her again. Then there was a speech therapist. She was DISMAL!!! When I asked why she was doing a certain thing she said that she was getting me ready to go back to work. I asked her if she knew what I did. She said no. I told her that I did corporate communications and change management for banks and insurance companies. I asked her if she knew what this was and she said no. I called Ryan and asked him if I could come back to him, but of course he said no. I was now an outpatient. My speech improved rapidly because I had friends to talk to instead of being in a room with a 93-year-old roommate.

My friend Judy K. was a Godsend! When I was released from Bridgepoint Judy was home on sick leave after an operation. She couldn't drive her car, but she could take transit. Twice a week she came to my house and took me out walking. I took out my coat and put it on. Then I finally realized that I couldn't wear it because it took two hands to do it up. Luckily, I had another coat which did up with snaps, which I could close with one hand. I went to put on my gloves, but my right hand was so swollen, it wouldn't fit in my gloves or mitts! Never-the-less we set off. We walked from my apartment (Avenue Road and St. Clair) to St. Clair and Yonge. I was terrified! I walked VERY slowly and constantly watched the pavement. Until Judy and I went out for this walk, the only walk that I'd been on was from Bridgepoint to the coffee shop and back. This walk was a whole lot longer! Without Judy, I don't know how I would have walked again. I was too afraid to go out walking alone. If you're recovering from a stroke, **PLEASE** ask a friend or family member to come and take you out walking until you have the confidence to go out on your own.

Some days Judy came to meet me at Shirley's at Toronto Rehab. We went to a breakfast place and I had bacon and eggs. I got good at cutting food with one hand. What an excitement! From there we walked to the Eaton Centre. It was very exciting for me to be out and about with tons of people! At the Eaton Centre I was looking for sneakers with NO laces and boots with NO laces – I only had one hand! I bought a pair of Sketcher's sneakers with no laces that needed to be tied and Judy convinced me to buy Blundstone's – the BEST boots I've ever had. When the salesperson brought them to me and looked at Judy and asked her if these were my style. She just looked at me and told me to buy them. Judy was absolutely right! I wear them winter,

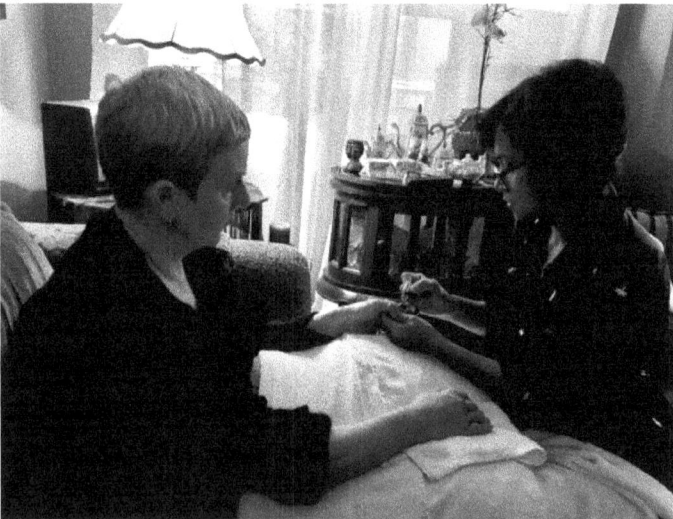

Judy arranged for a person to come to my house and give us both manicures and pedicures. It was wonderful!!! That's the Chanel nail polish colour that Teresa and Erin sent me.

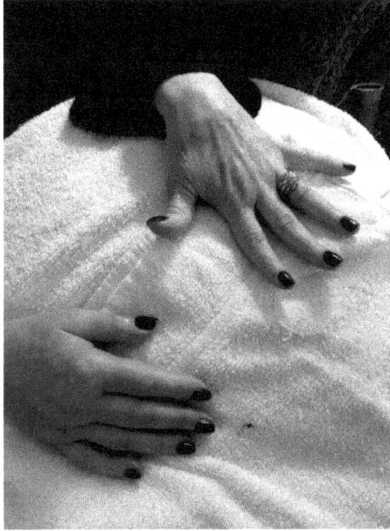

Look at how swollen my right hand still was! It was starting to move and
my occupational therapist was really pleased with my progress. I always did
my own manicures, but this wasn't going to work for me!
I found a place around the corner from my house that I could go to for
manicures and pedicures.

summer, spring and fall. I'll never be without a pair of Blundstone's
again. Thank you Judy!!!!

I've always been a member of the ROM (Royal Ontario Museum)
and the AGO (Art Gallery of Ontario), had theatre subscriptions,
tickets for concerts and subscriptions to the National Geographic Series
at Roy Thomson Hall. There were a few tickets that came up at the
end of November and the beginning of December, but I didn't feel that
I was ready to go. It was the stairs that scared the hell out of me, so I
gave my tickets away. Until I was comfortable, there was no sense in
going.

My mother was still at Toronto Rehab. The social worker said that
they had a really nice place – Hillcrest - that would be better for Shirley
and it was within walking distance from our apartments. Because I
believed the social worker, I agreed that Shirley would move. I went
with Shirley when she was transferred there. We almost had a heart

attack when we arrived! It was old and dumpy looking. We checked Shirley in to her room. It was a four-person room. Shirley didn't have any exercise because they didn't have a workout room. What was nice was that they had a dining room and it also had a television, so Shirley had people to talk to. But she had NOTHING that was going to make her any better. I called the social worker at the Toronto Rehab and asked her why she transferred Shirley to Hillcrest. The imbecile told me that she had never seen it! It finally occurred to me that the bitchy nurse that I had run ins with spoke to the social worker and had Shirley transferred. Mercifully in a few weeks Shirley started to feel very ill and they transferred her to Mount Sinai hospital where she was admitted. She would NEVER go back to Hillcrest again and she would NEVER go back to Toronto Rehab again. For rehab, Bridgepoint is the only place in Toronto that I would allow Shirley to be admitted to. Bridgepoint is the only place in Toronto that I would go or allow anyone that I know to go. It's a superb establishment! And they provide a quality of care like no one else!

The doctors at Mount Sinai were just wonderful to Shirley. Her cardiologist found the reasons that she had blown up and they were treating it. Within a few weeks, Shirley was down to her 128 pounds. Shirley knew in her heart that she didn't have a long life ahead and when she talked to her doctor about it, he agreed with her. He said she could have one to two years. When they started talking about sending her to rehab I told them why I only wanted her to go to Bridgepoint, gave them the reasons why, and they agreed. As a matter of fact, Bridgepoint is part of the Sinai Health System. Eventually, Shirley was sent to Bridgepoint. I was ecstatic! I could now see Shirley every day because I was at Bridgepoint two days a week for my outpatient therapy.

Shirley and I were very pleased with Bridgepoint. She had a beautiful room and a very lovely roommate who was around the same age as Shirley. The two of them were talking so much that neither of them needed a television which was wonderful, because when I was a Bridgepoint the televisions never worked! They had a beautiful workout room on her floor and she had a physiotherapist that came to take her every day for exercise. Shirley wasn't so crazy about the food so every once in a while I went downstairs and brought her a treat.

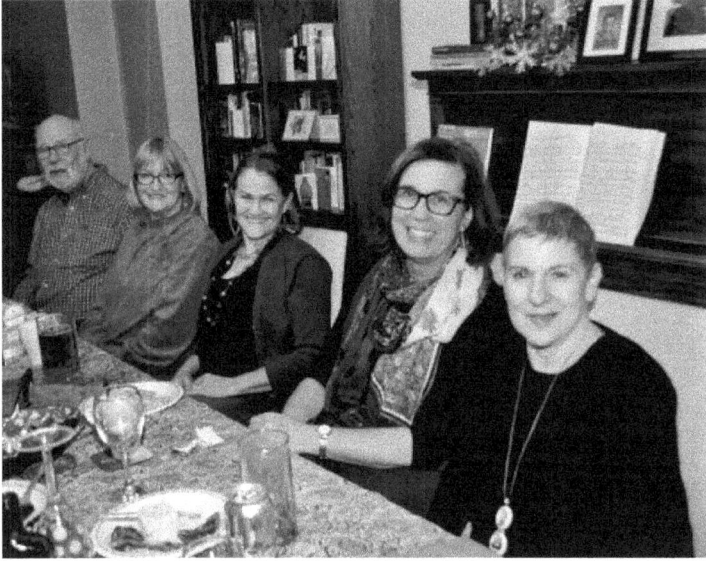

Cousin Bill, Cousin Abbie, Sue, Cousin Lisa & Me.

Time was moving quickly! And I was getting stronger every day! I spent Christmas with Sue's family. I'm part of Sue's family and she's part of mine.

Christmas dinner was wonderful! It was wonderful to be out of the hospital and rehab and working at outpatient therapy.

New Year's Eve I was back at Sue's and it was great! The house was full of friends. Thomas (Sue's son) was so attentive. Thomas, who was now 14 years old, knew I was afraid of the stairs. When I had to go to the bathroom upstairs and I got up to go, Thomas said, "Auntie Geri, please let me go up with you. I'll wait for you to finish and we'll go down together." I said, "Thank you Thomas" and we went together. He was wonderful! I left at about 10:00pm because I wake up around 5:00am regardless of what time I go to sleep. I couldn't wait to go to bed and see 2018 end and I start off a new year! YEAH! 2019!

Chapter 4
St. Anne's Spa in Grafton

It was now January 2019 and I was greatly improved! I was walking really well – thanks to Judy K.. My speech was improving! Look at the picture of me at St. Anne's Spa. My face is still partially paralyzed but I'm wearing MAC's Russian Red lipstick, blush and mascara! Yeah!!!!

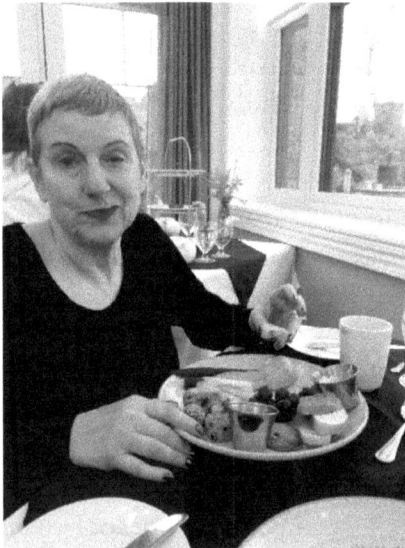

January 8, 2019.

My right hand was really less swollen and I had a manicure every two weeks.

Sue and I really had no intentions of going to St. Anne's. Sue had a great idea that we could get a really good deal to go to Cuba. I said that I should call and find out about getting travel insurance. I had a medical/dental plan that included travel insurance, so I called them. Of course I had to tell them that I had a stroke in September and the woman started almost yelling at me. She made it very clear that I couldn't travel for one year!!!! That did all the plans for Cuba. Sue did some checking around and found us a great deal at St. Anne's. There was no room in the hotel but we got a 4 bedroom house all to ourselves and we went to the hotel for food and our spa treatments.

We were at St. Anne's for two full days and one night. The spa treatments were absolutely luxurious! And the food was wonderful! It was a wonderful two days!

Our 4-Bedroom House.

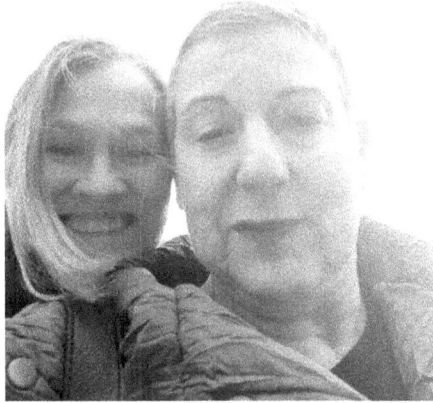

Our Selfie at St. Anne's Spa.

Chapter 5
Geri Versus The Ministry Of Transportation

This is the story of Geri versus The Ministry of Transportation. It goes on for FOUR MONTHS! I know that it breaks with the pattern of the story, but this is the way it goes. At the end of the story in May, we'll go back to February 2019.

When I had my stroke, it was immediately reported to the Ministry of Transportation. They sent me a letter saying that my Driver's License was suspended until which time **a doctor could verify that I was fit to drive**. At the end of January, I asked Dr. Heather MacNeil (my doctor at Bridgepoint) if she thought I could get my Driver's License back. And she said SURE THING!!!! She would have my occupational therapist do the tests (it take two hours) and then she would fill in the rest and send it to the Ministry of Transportation.

This is a timeline of my attempts to have my driving license reinstated:

Ministry of Transportation

September 12, 2018
I had a stroke and was taken to St. Mike's Hospital. This led to my driving license being suspended by the Ministry of Transport. As I recovered, I was transferred to Bridgepoint Healthcare.

January 24, 2019

After a lot of hard work, my doctor Heather MacNeill (at Bridgepoint Healthcare) ordered my tests and filled out the papers to get my license reinstated. She's done tons of these before as her patients are stroke survivors.

February 7 to April 2, 2019

The Ministry of Transportation has 30 days to answer your questions. On February 7, 2019 I received a letter from the Ministry of Transport asking three questions that were already answered in my application. My doctor was not amused but answered the questions on March 6, 2019. On March 26, 2019 the Ministry of Transportation sent a letter saying that my license was still under suspension with no reason why and asking for my significant improvement on my condition. On April 2, 2019 my doctor wrote a medical report saying that I was back to normal, she has no concerns about my returns to driving and that she "would advocate for a reinstatement of my license without the need for an on-road driver's test."

April 29 to May 1, 2019

On April 29, 2019 I called the Ministry of Transportation to find out why my license was still under suspension. I was talking to a woman named Rosalie who asked to put me on hold while she read my file. After five minutes she came back on the line and said, "I can't believe you don't have your license. I'll talk to my supervisor and get back to you within 48 hours." I NEVER heard back.

May 9 to May 10, 2019

On May 9, 2019 I called the Ministry of Transportation because I hadn't heard from them within 30 days. Valerie told me that they hadn't received my doctor's medical report. She asked me to email it in. I did. On May 9, 2019 I received an email saying that they received it and that it would now take between 10-15 days (or maybe longer) to review.

On May 10, 2019 I called the Ministry of Transportation to find out why my case couldn't be reviewed sooner. Valerie checked my file and told me that my doctor's medical report wasn't there. She asked for my email address and found my email and was now going to ask someone to file it. I asked if my file could be reviewed sooner and she said that she had no authority to order it.

Appeals Tribunal

On April 6, 2019 I filled out a file for the Appeals Tribunal because I was treated unfairly. My doctor said that I should have had my license back. Rosalie at the Ministry of Transportation said that I should have my license back. I sent the file Express Post that requires a signature. They signed on April 9, 2019. I called the Appeals Tribunal on May 10, 2019 and they said that they never received the file – which they signed for. I've given them the date that they signed for it and now I'm waiting.

I have never seen two government bodies so completely incompetent!

Called My Lawyer

I finally called my lawyer. I knew that I had no chance to bring a suit against the Ministry of Transportation, but I thought maybe he had an idea. The first thing he said was, "Go see your MPP (Member of Provincial Parliament)". As desperate as I was, the next morning at 10am, Sue and I walked into Jill Andrew's office. A young man, Phillip Morgan, greeted me. And lucky as I was, he's the person in the office who works the cases. I brought all of the paperwork with me and Phillip made photocopies.

Phillip said that he would call their liaison at the Ministry of Transportation that day and get back to me tomorrow. Instead of calling me tomorrow, he called me later that day and said that I would have my license back in 14 days. After four months of waiting for my license, I really didn't have faith that this would work, but I waited 14 days. Phillip called on the 14th day to say that **I HAD MY LICENSE BACK AND THAT I COULD DRIVE TODAY**. I started to cry... I'd waited four months and Phillip did in 14 days what my doctor couldn't do in four months. The very next day I DROVE to the LCBO and bought a very nice bottle of red wine and brought it to Phillip.

I was now engaged in trying to get the Deputy Registrar of Motor Vehicles fired! For four months he ignored my doctor (who treats only stroke patients), but when someone higher up at the Ministry of Transportation saw my files, he had no choice but to give me my license back. I filed complaints with the Ontario Ombudsman and with the Ministry of Transportation.

Thank you to Jill Andrew's MPP's office!!! Phillip Morgan got my license back for me. If you have any trouble with the Ministry of Transportation, call your MPP. Jill Andrew, as long as you're running to be my MPP, you'll get my vote.

A few weeks later I got a call from someone at the Ministry of Transportation who deals with problems with the institution. I explained the whole situation to him and he asked me what I wanted. I told him that I wanted the Deputy Registrar of Motor Vehicles fired. He explained to me that the Deputy Registrar of Motor Vehicles works for the government, so he couldn't get fired. Can you believe this idiocy!!!! He also told me that because his signature was on the papers that he sent me, he probably didn't even write them. One of his direct reports probably did. He said the best that he could do was offer them further training. And he thought he was being nice by giving me his email address in case I had further problems! He's the last person that I'd call!

I also got a call from the Ontario Ombudsman's office. She wanted to know what I wanted. I told her the same thing that I told the Ministry of Transportation – I wanted the Deputy Registrar of Motor Vehicles fired. I told her the whole story. She told me that because my case had now been settled, they couldn't do a thing, except for leaving my case open in case there was another one similar. Again, I couldn't get anything done!!!

Sue actually had the best explanation. Most people don't start to get better after a stroke for about one year. My doctor applied for my license reinstatement after 4 ½ months. Sue was convinced that the Deputy Registrar of Motor Vehicles would have continued to refuse me until I had hit one year. Ladies and gentlemen, if you have problems getting your license reinstated, call your MPP!!! And if you're looking for a job that you can't get fired from, go work for the government!

Chapter 6
No More Therapy

My outpatient therapy continued until February 14, 2019. After all the work that I did, my right hand began moving! The more I used it, the swelling started to very slowly disappear. My occupational therapist said that she'd never seen a patient recover so quickly. I still continued doing my workout program that I started in November. I also had my last visit with a physical therapist. My physical therapist was taking six months off and doing exotic travelling. I had a physical therapist that I knew when I was an in patient at Bridgepoint. She gave me my last treatment and suggested that I look into yoga. I loved yoga and had done it before, so I'd be sure to check it out. I had two sessions left with the speech therapist and I said "no thanks." She asked me if I was ready to go back to work. Of course, I said yes. She didn't believe me so she called my friend Sue and asked her. Of course, she said yes! Before I left they gave me an appointment with Dr. Heather MacNeill for April.

I was getting stronger. I was now drinking smoothies again because I HAD TWO HANDS!!!!!!!!!!!!!! You have no idea how wonderful life is with two hands that are working. I was back to cooking – no more microwaved food! And I was typing with two hands. I had a lot of work to do on my right hand, arm and leg, but I was ready!

I was back to the theatre! I still really didn't like the stairs, but I could navigate them. I was reclaiming my life!

Judy K. started me off walking, but I had to continue to get myself back to 10 kms/day. I continued walking from my apartment to Yonge St.. When that became easy, I walked south on Yonge St. to Summerhill and back. That was difficult because going south on Yonge St. was easy because it was downhill but coming back up was a challenge. But, I was made for challenges! I continued down Yonge St. past Summerhill to Rosedale. And then to Bloor. Yeah! I now knew that I could walk anywhere!

I made sure that I walked several hours per day. If the weather wasn't nice I had a stair machine. I bought it years ago so that I could walk every day.

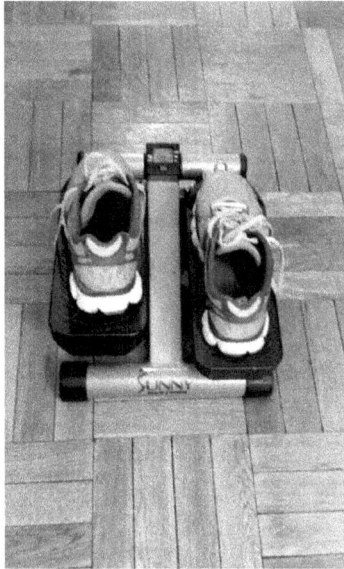

My Stair Machine.

The problem was that the Stair Machine had no frame. It was never a problem before, but now I didn't have a good sense of balance, so I couldn't be on it for very long. But, I persevered. Every day I added a few more minutes until I could walk for one hour without getting off. Between walking outdoors and on my Stair Machine, by March I was up to 10 kms/day. I was starting to feel LIKE ME!

In March Shirley came home from rehab. She was certainly better than she'd been, but Shirley really wasn't herself. A nurse came in to see her three times per week to change the bandages on her legs and a personal support worker also came in three times per week to give her a bath. Both of these people were lovely and Shirley really enjoyed them. The reality was that Shirley really couldn't walk without her walker. Shirley sat in the living room and watched the cooking shows on TV during the day and Judge Judy in the evening. I came up every day and made dinner for us. Then I cleaned up and we watched something else on TV after Judge Judy and then I put her to bed. Every morning I went up at 7:00am to check on her and I went up in the afternoon too.

One day Shirley shocked me! She told me that she just wanted to live long enough to see me recover from my stroke and to attend my 65th birthday party. "What birthday party? You know I've never liked birthday parties." I said. Shirley looked at me and said, "You're going to make yourself a birthday party." I couldn't refuse Shirley anything, so I figured I'd plan something later.

In March my friend Debbie from Montreal came in for the day with her husband who came in for business – lucky me! Debbie and I have been friends since we were nine years old. We met at Pine Valley Summer Camp in the Laurentians (I was a camper there with Debbie from '63 – '70 and it was FABULOUS!!!). Two years later my parents moved us to Ville St. Laurent and I walked into my new Grade 6 class and there was Debbie! We were friends ever since. Debbie and I met at the Eaton Centre. Of course I walked because I was now walking 10 kms/day. We had a fabulous lunch and walked and talked and talked and talked. What a super day!!

Sonya
One of the things I love to do with Geri, besides shopping, is eating good food in Toronto. I remember very clearly having brunch with her at La Société in March 2019, just 6 months after her stroke. We had lobster eggs benedict! Sitting across from her I couldn't help but be amazed at her recovery. The symptoms of aphasia were barely there and she had regained almost full dexterity in her right hand. I don't think

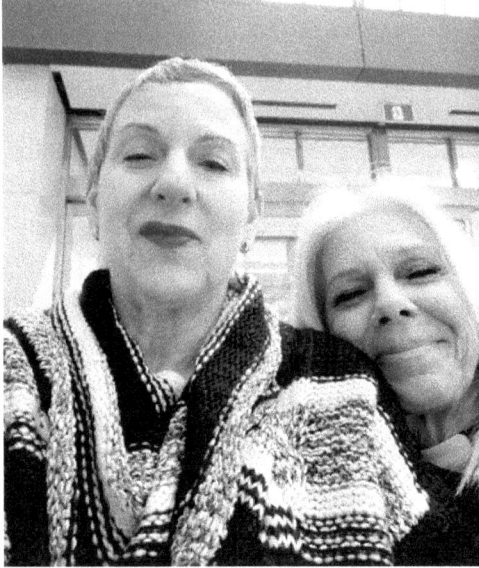

March 2019.
Me and Debbie—Our Selfie in the Eaton Centre.

anyone who hadn't know her before that day could have suspected she suffered a life-threatening stroke only 6 months ago. I continue to be amazed 'til this day.

Geri

Sue had a brilliant idea for a new business – Memorable Lives. Every family has stories to tell and memories to share. At memorablelives.ca she creates beautiful, one-of-a-kind family history books that capture life stories and preserve your memories for future generations. She asked Shirley if she'd like to participate and have a book written about her. Shirley was very excited as long as she could tell the story that she wanted to tell – her love story with Joe. Sue and Shirley worked together for weeks.

Sue

I had been let go from my job at the bank and had been thinking about a change in direction. I did some career counselling and came up with the idea for Memorable Lives, combining my love of history and writing. I needed a demo book and thought about asking Shirley. Much to my delight Shirley was up for it and between Geri and Shirley we had lots of photos to use. I would come up with my dog Kyser, who Shirley loved. Shirley would tell me "we have work to do" and so we did. We would chat for about an hour and I would take notes. As the book grew, Shirley got to review it. It was fascinating for me to learn about her life story. It was truly a love affair with her husband Joe from their teenage years till his death.

Geri

In April I went back to Bridgepoint to visit with Dr. Heather MacNeill. She had a resident with her. He had read my chart and then looked at me and then turned to Dr. MacNeill and asked, "Is this her?" Dr. MacNeill said, "Yes." He turned to me, just stunned! Dr. MacNeill asked if we could make an appointment in June and I said, "Of course." I knew that would be my last appointment with Dr. MacNeill and I would be very sad to say good-bye.

Chapter 7: Are You at Risk for A Stroke?

A stroke can strike anyone at any age!

Each year, 15 million people worldwide suffer a stroke, according to World Health Organisation statistics. From this number, about five million die, while another five million experience a permanent disability including paralysis, speech difficulty, loss of sight and confusion.

What is a stroke? A stroke happens when blood stops flowing to any part of your brain, damaging brain cells. The effects of a stroke depend on the part of the brain that was damaged and the amount of damage done.

According to the Heart & Stroke Foundation:
The brain is full of specialized cells called neurons. These neurons make the brain work. To work properly — and even to survive — they need to be fed by a constant supply of blood. To survive, vessels need to be fed by a constant supply of blood.

Blood vessels of the brain: Arteries and veins are types of blood vessels in your body. Arteries carry blood, rich in oxygen and nutrients, to your organs. Veins carry waste products away from your organs. Cerebral arteries are the arteries of the brain. Normal brain function needs a constant supply of oxygen and nutrients.

When a stroke happens, the blood flow is disrupted. Some brain cells do not get the oxygen and nutrients they need. When the cells die, that area of the brain cannot function as it did before.

What are the effects of a stroke? The effects of stroke are different for each person. They can be mild, moderate or severe. The severity depends on factors such as:
- Type of stroke (ischemic or hemorrhagic)
- Side of the brain where the stroke occurred (right or left hemisphere)
- Regions of the brain affected by the stroke
- Size of the damaged area in the brain
- Body functions controlled by the affected area
- Amount of time the brain area had no blood flow
- Time it took to get to hospital to receive treatment

"Strokes can happen to anyone, anywhere, anytime." according to Dr. Kara Sands from the Mayo Clinic. Anyone from infants to the elderly can have a stroke. But the risk of stroke doubles for each decade between the ages of 55 and 85. And, strokes are the world's leading cause of disability and the second most cause of death. Dr. Kara Sands says that 80% of strokes are preventable with lifestyle changes! "Strokes are preventable, treatable and beatable as long as you think fast."

For strokes in young people, the most common symptoms of stroke are loss of speech, facial droop and weakness on one side of the body. They are the same in younger patients as those who are older. Other symptoms can include vision loss, double vision, slurred speech, dizziness, or difficulty walking. Identifying stroke as a cause for these symptoms is often delayed by a lack of recognition that stroke can happen to young people. About 10% - 15% of strokes occur in children and adults under age 45, and that number is rising.

Did you know that... According to the Heart and Stroke Foundation, stroke can happen to anyone, at any age. Yet stroke disproportionately affects women – more women die of stroke, women have worse outcomes after stroke, more women are living with the effects of stroke and women face more challenges as they recover.

Women's bodies are not the same as men's and stroke affects them differently at different stages of life. The risk of stroke is higher during pregnancy. As women's bodies adapt to menopause, stroke risk increases again. Elderly women are especially vulnerable: they are the most likely to have a stroke; their strokes are the most severe; their outcomes are the poorest; and stroke can put an end to their independence.

Can a healthy person have a stroke? Anyone can have a stroke, but some things put you at higher risk. And some things can lower your risk. If you're 55 and older, if you're African-American, if you're a man, or if you have a family history of strokes or heart attacks, your chances of having a stroke are higher.

Strokes can be classified into 2 main categories:
Ischemic strokes: About 87% of all strokes are ischemic. This is the most common type of stroke. It happens when the brain's blood vessels become narrowed or blocked, causing severely reduced blood flow (ischemia). Blocked or narrowed blood vessels are caused by fatty deposits that build up in blood vessels or by blood clots or other debris that travel through the bloodstream, most often from the heart, and lodge in the blood vessels in the brain. Some initial research shows that COVID-19 infection may increase the risk of ischemic stroke, but more study is needed.

Hemorrhagic strokes: These are strokes caused by bleeding. About 13% of all strokes are hemorrhagic. Hemorrhagic stroke occurs when a blood vessel in the brain leaks or ruptures. Brain hemorrhages can result from many conditions that affect the blood vessels. Factors related to hemorrhagic stroke include:

- Uncontrolled high blood pressure
- Over treatment with blood thinners (anticoagulants)
- Bulges at weak spots in your blood vessel walls (aneurysms)
- Trauma (such as a car accident)

- Protein deposits in blood vessel walls that lead to weakness in the vessel wall (cerebral amyloid angiopathy)
- Ischemic stroke leading to hemorrhage

Beware of TIA (Transient Ischemic Attack) or Mini-Stroke

TIAs are sometimes known as "warning strokes." It is important to know that:

- A TIA is a warning sign of a future stroke.
- A TIA is a medical emergency, just like a major stroke.
- Strokes and TIAs require emergency care. Call 9-1-1 right away if you feel signs of a stroke or see symptoms in someone around you.
- There is no way to know in the beginning whether symptoms are from a TIA or from a major type of stroke.
- Like ischemic strokes, blood clots often cause TIAs.
- More than a third of people who have a TIA and don't get treatment have a major stroke within 1 year. As many as 10% to 15% of people will have a major stroke within 3 months of a TIA.

Recognizing and treating TIAs can lower the risk of a major stroke! If your stroke symptoms go away after a few minutes, you may have had a transient ischemic attack (TIA).. Although brief, a TIA is a sign of a serious condition that will not go away without medical help. Unfortunately, because TIAs clear up, many people ignore them. But paying attention to a TIA can save your life. If you think you or someone you know has had a TIA, tell a health care team about the symptoms right away.

Brain Stem Strokes

When stroke occurs in the brain stem, depending on the severity of the injury, it can affect both sides of the body and may leave someone in a 'locked-in' state. When a locked-in state occurs, the patient is generally unable to speak or achieve any movement below the neck.

According to the American Heart Association brain stem strokes can have complex symptoms, and they can be difficult to diagnose. A person may have vertigo, dizziness and severe imbalance without the hallmark of most strokes — weakness on one side of the body. The symptoms of vertigo dizziness or imbalance usually occur together; dizziness alone is not a sign of stroke. A brain stem stroke can also cause double vision, slurred speech and decreased consciousness.

Only a half-inch in diameter, the brain stem controls all basic activities of the central nervous system: consciousness, blood pressure and breathing. All motor control for the body flows through it. Brain stem strokes can impair any or all of these functions. More severe brain stem strokes can cause locked-in syndrome, a condition in which survivors can move only their eyes.

If a stroke in the brain stem results from a clot, the faster blood flow can be restored, the better the chances for recovery. Patients should receive treatment as soon as possible for the best recovery.

Like all strokes, brain stem strokes produce a wide spectrum of deficits and recovery. Whether a survivor has minor or severe deficits depends on the location of the stroke within the brain stem, the extent of injury and how quickly treatment is provided.

Risk factors for brain stem stroke are the same as for strokes in other areas of the brain: high blood pressure, diabetes, heart disease, atrial fibrillation and smoking Similarly, brain stem strokes can be caused by a clot or a hemorrhage. There are also rare causes, like injury to an artery due to sudden head or neck movements.

Recovery is possible. Because brain stem strokes do not usually affect language ability, the patient is often able to participate more fully in rehabilitation. Double vision and vertigo usually resolve after several weeks of recovery in mild to moderate brain stem strokes.

The Hemispheres of the Brain

The brain is divided into two parts called hemispheres, the right and the left. The right hemisphere of your brain controls the left side of your body. The left hemisphere of your brain controls the right side of your body. Some functions are controlled by both. This picture by the Heart & Stroke Foundation shows the functions of the two hemispheres of the brain.

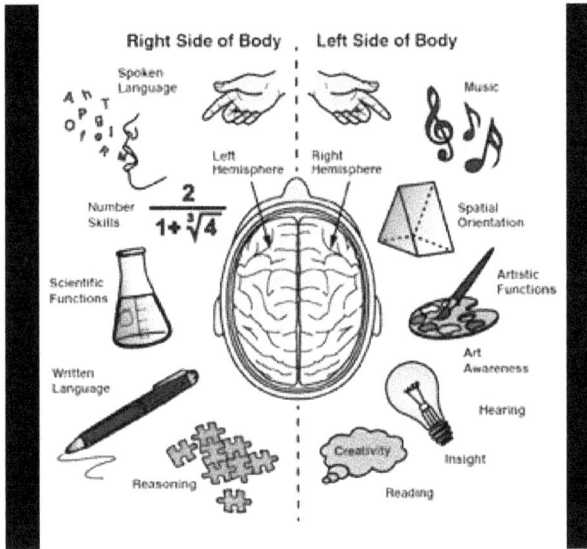

Right Side of Body . **Left Side of Body**

If you look at what the left hemisphere controls, then you know for sure that my stroke was in my left hemisphere! I couldn't talk and the right side of my body was paralyzed.

Other factors associated with a higher risk of stroke include:

- **Age** — People age 55 or older have a higher risk of stroke than do younger people.
- **Race or ethnicity** — African Americans and Hispanics have a higher risk of stroke than do people of other races or ethnicities.
- **Sex** — Men have a higher risk of stroke than do women. Women are usually older when they have strokes, and they're more likely to die of strokes than are men.
- **Hormones** — Use of birth control pills or hormone therapies that include estrogen increases risk.

What treatment is used for stroke? The main treatment for an ischemic stroke is a medicine called **tissue plasminogen activator (tPA)**. These thrombolytic drugs are often called **clot busters**. tPA is short for tissue plasminogen activator and can only be given to patients who are having a stroke caused by a blood clot (ischemic stroke). It can stop a stroke by breaking up the blood clot. It breaks up the blood clots that block blood flow to your brain. This type of medicine must be given within 3 hours after your symptoms start. I was treated with a clot buster and I believe that I reached the hospital within 2.5 hours of my stroke.

How likely is a second stroke? Even after surviving a stroke, you're not out of the woods, since having one makes it a lot more likely that you'll have another. In fact, of the 795,000 Americans who will have a first stroke this year, **23 percent** will suffer a second stroke.

You can reverse your stroke risk by taking care of:

- **High blood pressure**: It's the most treatable stroke risk factor.
- **Smoking**: People who smoke are two to four times more likely to have a stroke.
- **Diabetes**: Increases your risk of having a stroke.
- **Atrial Fibrillation**: It increases stroke by five to seven times.
- **High Cholesterol**: With too much bad cholesterol, it turns to plaque which clogs arteries and causes strokes by blood clots.
- **Binge drinking**: Can lead to a stroke.
- **Physical inactivity and obesity**: They increase strokes by three times. Always see your doctor regularly. The doctor can check for silent stroke (is a stroke without any noticeable symptoms) risk factors and help you manage any chronic illnesses.

How do you know if you're having a stroke?

If you're lucky enough that you haven't just passed out, remember the word **FAST** and call 911.

FAST stands for:

F: Face – Is it drooping?

A: Arms – Can you raise both?
S: Speech – Is it slurred or jumbled?
T: Time – Time to call 911 right away!

Preventive Medications: If you've had an ischemic stroke or a TIA, your doctor may recommend medications to help reduce your risk of having another stroke. These include:

> • **Anti-platelet drugs.** Platelets are cells in the blood that form clots. Anti-platelet drugs make these cells less sticky and less likely to clot.

> • **Anticoagulants.** These drugs reduce blood clotting. Several newer blood-thinning medications (anticoagulants) are available for preventing strokes in people who have a high risk. These medications include dabigatran (Pradaxa), rivaroxaban (Xarelto), apixaban (Eliquis) and edoxaban (Savaysa). They're shorter acting than warfarin and usually don't require regular blood tests or monitoring by your doctor. These drugs are also associated with a lower risk of bleeding complications compared to warfarin. I'm taking dabigatran (Pradaxa).

What disabilities can result from a stroke? According to **The National Institute of Neurological Disorders and Stroke** the types and degrees of disability that follow a stroke depend upon which area of the brain is damaged. Generally, a stroke can cause five types of disabilities: **Paralysis or problems controlling movement (motor control)** Damage to cells and connections in the brain following a stroke can cause various problems with movement and sensation, including:

> • Paralysis, loss of voluntary movement, or weakness that usually affects one side of the body, usually the side opposite to the side damaged by the stroke (such as the face, an arm, a leg, or the entire side of the body). Paralysis on one side of the body is called *hemiplegia*; weakness on one side is called *hemiparesis*.

> • Problems swallowing (*dysphagia*)

• Loss of control of body movements, including problems with body posture, walking, and balance (*ataxia*)

Sensory disturbances, including pain Several sensory disturbances can develop following a stroke, including:

• Losing the ability to feel touch, pain, temperature, or sense how the body is positioned. People who had a stroke also could lose the ability to recognize objects that they are holding or even their own limb.

• Pain, numbness, a feeling of heaviness in a limb, or odd sensations such as tingling or prickling in a paralyzed or weakened limb (called *paresthesia*). Numbness or tingling in a limb may continue even after recovering some movement.

• Loss of bladder and bowel control and loss of mobility to reach a toilet in time. Permanent incontinence after a stroke is uncommon.

• Chronic pain syndromes can occur as a result of mechanical problems caused by the weakness. Most often, the pain results from lack of movement in a joint that has been immobilized for a prolonged period of time (such as weakness or spasticity and the tendons and ligaments around the joint becoming fixed in one position). This is commonly called a "frozen" joint; treatment involves having a therapist or trained caregiver gently move or flex the joint to prevent painful "freezing" and to allow easy movement after voluntary motor strength returns.

More rarely pain can occur due to stroke-induced damage to the nervous system (neuropathic pain), the most common which is called "thalamic pain syndrome" (caused by a stroke to the thalamus, which processes sensory information from the body to the brain).

Problems using or understanding language (aphasia) At least one-fourth of all stroke survivors experience language impairments, involving the ability to speak, write, and understand spoken and written language. In right-handed individuals these strokes usually involve the left side of the brain. A stroke-induced injury to any of the brain's language-control centers can severely impair verbal communication. There are several types of aphasia:

> • *expressive aphasia*, in which people lose the ability to speak or write the words they are thinking and to put words together in coherent, grammatically correct sentences.

> • *receptive aphasia*, in which people have difficulty understanding spoken or written language and often have incoherent speech. Although these individuals can form grammatically correct sentences, their utterances are often devoid of meaning.

> • *global aphasia*, in which people lose nearly all their linguistic abilities; they cannot understand language or use it to convey thought.

Problems with thinking and memory Strokes can damage the parts of the brain responsible for memory, learning, and awareness. A stroke survivor may have a dramatically shortened attention span or may experience deficits in short-term memory. Some people also may lose the ability to make plans, comprehend meaning, learn new tasks, or engage in other complex mental activities. Common deficits resulting from stroke are:

> • *anosognosia*, an inability to acknowledge the reality of the physical impairments resulting from a stroke.

> • *neglect*, the loss of the ability to respond to objects or sensory stimuli located on the stroke-impaired side. This most commonly affects the left side of people with stroke on the right side of their brain.

> • *apraxia*, the loss of ability to carry out a learned purposeful movement or to plan the steps involved in a complex task and act on them in the proper sequence. People with apraxia also may have problems following instructions.

Emotional disturbances After a stroke someone might feel fear, anxiety, frustration, anger, sadness, and a sense of grief over physical and mental losses. Some emotional disturbances and personality changes are caused by the physical effects of brain damage. Clinical depression—a sense of hopelessness that disrupts the ability to function—is commonly experienced by stroke survivors. Post-stroke depression can be treated with antidepressant medications and psychological counseling.

Talk about how you feel with your healthcare team. Your doctor may recommend steps you can take.

> • **Joining a patient support group** may help you adjust to life after a stroke. You can see how other people manage similar symptoms and their condition. Talk with your doctor about local support groups or check with an area medical center.

> • **Medicines, such as antidepressants,** or other treatments can improve your quality of life.

> • **Support from family and friends** can help relieve stress and anxiety. Let your loved ones know how you feel and what they can do to help you.

Learn the warning signs of serious complications

The most common side effect of taking blood thinners to reduce your stroke risk is bleeding. This happens if the medicine thins your blood too much. This side effect can be life-threatening. Bleeding can occur inside your body cavities or from the surface of your skin.

Know the warning signs of bleeding so you can get help right away. They include:

- Blood in your urine, bright red blood in your stools, or black tarry stools

- Bright red vomit or vomit that looks like coffee grounds

- Increased menstrual flow

- Pain in your abdomen or severe pain in your head

- Unexplained bleeding from the gums and nose

- Unexplained bruising or tiny red or purple dots on the skin

Easy bruising or bleeding may mean that your blood is too thin. Call your doctor right away if you have any of these signs. If you have severe bleeding, call 9-1-1.

Stroke Statistics According to the CDC (Centers for Disease Control and Prevention)

- In 2020, 1 in 6 deaths from cardiovascular disease was due to stroke.

- Every 40 seconds, someone in the United States has a stroke. Every 3.5 minutes, someone dies of stroke.

- Every year, more than 795,000 people in the United States have a stroke. About 610,000 of these are first or new strokes.

- About 185,000 strokes—nearly 1 in 4—are in people who have had a previous stroke.

- About 87% of all strokes are , in which blood flow to the brain is blocked.

- Stroke-related costs in the United States came to nearly $53 billion between 2017 and 2018. This total includes the cost of health care services, medicines to treat stroke, and missed days of work.

- Stroke is a leading cause of serious long-term disability.[2] Stroke reduces mobility in more than half of stroke survivors age 65 and older.

Stroke statistics by race and ethnicity

• Stroke is a leading cause of death for Americans, but the risk of having a stroke varies with race and ethnicity.

• Risk of having a first stroke is nearly twice as high for Blacks as for Whites, and Blacks have the highest rate of death due to stroke.

• Though stroke death rates have declined for decades among all race/ethnicities, Hispanics have seen an increase in death rates since 2013.

Stroke risk varies by age

• Stroke risk increases with age, but strokes can—and do—occur at any age.

• In 2014, 38% of people hospitalized for stroke were less than 65 years old.

Early action is important for stroke. Know the warning of stroke so that you can act fast if you or someone you know might be having a stroke. The chances of survival are greater when emergency treatment begins quickly.

• In one survey, most respondents—93%—recognized sudden numbness on one side as a symptom of stroke. Only 38% were aware of all major symptoms and knew to call 9-1-1 when someone was having a stroke.

• Patients who arrive at the emergency room within 3 hours of their first symptoms often have less disability 3 months after a stroke than those who received delayed care.

Live healthy, be active and live smoke free.

Chapter 8 – Stroke Recovery & Support

I am **EXTRAORDINARILY LUCKY** that I **fully** recovered from a life-threatening stroke!!! But if you ask anyone that knows me, they will tell you that I fully recovered because I worked harder than anyone else. Even though I believe that's true, I still feel that I'm EXTRAORDINARILY LUCKY to be part of a handful of stroke patients that are 100 percent recovered!

See the following statistics. According to the National Stroke Association, 10 percent of people who have a stroke recover **almost** completely – and **I recovered 100%**, with 25 percent recovering with minor impairments. Another 40 percent experience moderate to severe impairments that require special care. This means that there is a type of disability that affects your daily function, whether at work or in your personal life. And 10 percent require long-term care in a nursing home or other facility.

Can a person live alone while they are recovering from a stroke? Yes! I did! You can be as independent as possible. Often this means adding special equipment like grab bars or transfer benches. For your safety, you may need to have handrails installed in your bathroom. I also needed a shower bench and a three-step bench to get into bed. And I had a Phillips Lifeline in case I fell, it would check in with me first and if I didn't respond, it would call 911.

Successful stroke recovery depends on a number of factors, including:

- How much damage the stroke caused

- How soon recovery is started

- How high your motivation is and how hard you work toward recovery – I was highly motivated and I worked as hard as I could each and every day!!

- Your age when it happened

- Whether you have other medical problems that can affect recover

Some of the **residual effects of a stroke** that patients may have include:

- Difficulty with memory, thinking, awareness, attention, learning, and judgment

- Difficulty with speaking or understanding speech

- Trouble controlling or expressing emotions

- Bladder and bowel control issues

- Paralysis, weakness, or numbness (or all three) on one side

- Extremity pain, especially in the hands or feet and especially in cold weather

- Difficulty with chewing or swallowing

- Depression and anxiety

How the Brain Heals Itself

Our brains are amazing! They have the ability to re-wire itself, allowing us to improve skills such as walking, talking and using your affected arm. This process is known as neuroplasticity. It begins after a stroke, and it can continue for years. Neuroplasticity refers to the brain's ability to reorganize neurons in response to learning or experience.

Your brain is composed of over . These connections are pathways in your brain that retrieve and store information. When a stroke occurs, part of the brain becomes damaged and many of these connections are destroyed. That is why many patients struggle with mobility after a stroke, for example; because the neural connections that control movement have been compromised. However, through neuroplasticity, the brain can form new neural pathways. It can even transfer functions that were once held in damaged parts of the brain to new, healthy areas. This process allows you to regain movement and other skills after a stroke.

In the past, scientists believed that the adult brain was static. This meant that, after a certain point in development, the brain could no longer adapt to change. Today, however, that the brain is always in a flexible state, even in old age. This flexible state is called **plasticity**.

Research has also demonstrated that and cause changes in the brain. Therefore, a key aspect in stroke recovery is : exercises with high repetition. When you perform an action, your brain creates new neural pathways in response to your movement. These pathways make it easier for the brain to store and retrieve information. The more you practice that action, the more you reinforce those neural pathways, and the easier that activity becomes. This explains why the first time a person tries to play pickleball, they miss many or all shots. But by the hundredth time, they're hitting it like they always should. That's neuroplasticity in action. Therefore, to learn how to , you will need to practice speech therapy exercises several times a day. The same principle applies if you want to improve your balance, and even your memory. Whatever ability you want to improve, with enough practice, you will activate neuroplasticity and help your brain heal itself after stroke. Eventually, you should start to regain that function.

While neuroplasticity can help your brain heal itself after stroke, it also has a downside you should watch out for. Therapists call this phenomenon **maladaptive plasticity**. Maladaptive plasticity occurs when you consistently repeat an action **the wrong way**. For example, if you can't move your right hand to pick up a cup, you might start using your left hand instead. However, if you continue to only use your left hand, eventually your brain will "forget" how to use your right hand. This leads to a condition known as learned non-use, and it can lead to permanent loss of function. Therefore, if your right hand is weak, try to resist the urge to do everything with your left hand. Instead, try to use your right hand as much as you can, even if you have to give it a little assistance with the other hand. That's why my occupational therapist always told me that if there was something that I wanted to do with the right hand to **TRY**. And I did and I have my full mobility back! Of course it took months, but I did it.

By focusing on high repetition during stroke rehabilitation, you can activate neuroplasticity and help your brain heal itself after stroke. When you activate neuroplasticity through exercise, you help your brain repair lost connections. That not only lets you relearn certain activities, it also prevents neuronal decay and keeps your condition from deteriorating. Therefore, even if you have suffered a severe stroke, like I did, you can still make a functional recovery. Stay disciplined, work hard, and you will see results. **I did!**

Tips for a Healthy Diet to Help Stroke Recovery

According to the National Heart, Lung and Blood Institute (NIH):

- Vegetables such as leafy greens (spinach, collard greens, kale, cabbage), broccoli, and carrots

- Fruits such as apples, bananas, oranges, pears, grapes, and prunes

- Whole grains such as plain oatmeal, brown rice, and whole-grain bread or tortillas

- Fat-free or low-fat dairy foods such as milk, cheese, or yogurt

- Protein-rich foods:

o Fish high in omega-3 fatty acids (salmon, tuna, and trout)

- Lean meats such as 95% lean ground beef or pork tenderloin or skinless chicken or turkey

- Eggs

- Nuts, seeds, and soy products (tofu)

- Legumes such as kidney beans, lentils, chickpeas, black-eyed peas, and lima beans

- Oils and foods high in monounsaturated and polyunsaturated fats:

- Canola, corn, olive, safflower, sesame, sunflower, and soybean oils (not coconut or palm oil)

- Nuts such as walnuts, almonds, and pine nuts

- Nut and seed butters

- Salmon and trout

- Seeds (sesame, sunflower, pumpkin, or flax)

- Avocados

- Tofu

Foods to limit

A heart-healthy eating plan limits sodium (salt), saturated fat, added sugars, and alcohol. Understanding nutrition labels can help you choose healthier foods.

Limit sodium

Adults and children over age 14 should eat less than 2,300 milligrams of a day. Children younger than age 14 may need to eat even less sodium each day based on their sex and age. If you have , you may need to limit sodium even more. Talk to your healthcare provider about the amount of sodium that is right for you or your child.

Try these shopping and cooking tips to help you choose and prepare foods that are lower in sodium:

- **Read food labels** and choose products that have less sodium for the same serving size.

- **Choose low-sodium**, reduced-sodium, or no-salt-added products.

- **Choose fresh, frozen, or no-salt-added foods** instead of pre-seasoned, sauce-marinated, brined, or processed meats, poultry, and vegetables.

- **Eat at home more often** so you can cook food from scratch, which will allow you to control the amount of sodium in your meals.

- **Flavor foods with herbs and spices** instead of salt.

- **When cooking, limit your use of pre-made sauces, mixes, and instant products** such as rice, noodles, and ready-made pasta.

What is stroke rehabilitation? Stroke rehabilitation or "rehab" helps you regain as much independence and quality of life as possible. Rehab can help you physically, emotionally, socially and spiritually after stroke. It helps restore you to optimal health, functioning and well-being. Rehabilitate comes from the Latin "habilitas" which means "to make able again."

According to the Heart & Stroke Foundation, **rehabilitation is a process**. Rehabilitation should start as soon as possible after your stroke, typically while you are still in hospital and will continue after you leave. Rehabilitation can happen in many places: a specialized stroke rehabilitation unit in the hospital, a separate rehabilitation hospital, an outpatient rehabilitation centre or community program, and at home. The place where you receive your rehabilitation may change as you progress to best meet your needs and goals. You are at the centre of your plan at every step of your journey. Participation in outpatient rehabilitation following discharge from acute and/or rehabilitation inpatient services should be available and will help you continue to make gains toward your rehabilitation goals.

You are the most important part of the recovery. Work with your healthcare team to **develop a personalized plan to achieve your goals. Share what you want to accomplish during rehabilitation** and include this in the plan. The team should work with you to update your plan as you progress, so it always fits your current needs and improving abilities.

Tips for successful rehabilitation - **Practice, Practice, Practice**. To achieve the best recovery, it is important to **practice the exercises and activities** you are taught in your rehabilitation therapy sessions. The healthcare team should work with you and your family and caregivers to identify activities you can safely do on your own, between sessions. Be sure you understand their instructions. Ask questions until you do. Use technology to help! The power of community. If you have experienced stroke or heart condition, or are caring for someone who has, connecting with other people who know what you are going through can help the recovery journey. These communities share experiences, quality information and tips, while offering social and emotional support in a safe, inclusive and respectful community. Keep at it. Everyone's recovery from stroke is different. Rehabilitation and reintegration into the community will happen at your own pace. In some cases, improvement is not seen for weeks, months, or even years after the stroke occurred then new improvements can happen. Stay informed! Ask your healthcare team for a list of community resources on your transition to home.

Advocate. Rehabilitation therapy is important. If the stroke has affected your ability to walk, use your arms, think, see, or speak, you will need rehabilitation to help you recover. As much as possible, advocate on your own behalf for access to rehabilitation therapy.

Stroke rehabilitation is comprised of:

- **Speech therapy** helps people who have problems producing or understanding speech.
- **Physical therapy** uses exercises to help you relearn movement and coordination skills
you may have lost because of the stroke.
- **Occupational therapy** focuses on improving daily activities, such as eating, drinking, dressing, bathing, reading, and writing.

What type of rehab should you expect? Your rehab depends upon:

- how severe your stroke was
- the part of your brain that was affected
- the effects of the stroke on your body, mind and emotions
- your general health
- your ability to actively take part in your recovery
- your support system of family and caregivers

The medical experts who help you rehabilitate can also affect how well you recover and **mine were just superb!** I had the best speech therapist, physical therapist and occupational therapist. The more skilled they are, the better your recovery may be. Your family members and friends can also help improve your outlook by providing encouragement and support. Again, **mine were just superb!**

You can increase your chances of successfully recovering by practicing your rehabilitation exercises on a regular basis. **I did my home workouts seven days a week!** So, PLEASE do physical activities! They'll help you maintain a healthy weight, reduce high blood pressure, lower cholesterol levels, manage diabetes and manage stress and **it can significantly reduce your risk of heart disease and stroke**. Just like I talked to my occupational therapist and physical therapist, talk to your healthcare team about the right way for you to get active. No matter what your state of health is, there is something you can do to stay active. As I improved, I went back to walking. And after that I went back to yoga and then golf and I've recently taken up pickleball! There is something out there for you!

You'll see the fastest improvement in the weeks and up to six months right after the stroke. Progress slows between six months and a year, but if you continue to work at it, you may continue to see slower improvement over years.

After Stroke, Should You Do Exercise?

The best exercise after a stroke varies from person to person. Every stroke is different, and every patient sustains different secondary effects. This impacts the type of exercise that will be most beneficial for each patient. Therefore, every stroke survivor should talk to their therapist for the best recommendations.

According to FlintRehab, exercise after stroke is critical for two main reasons: rehabilitating the physical effects of a stroke and preventing another stroke from happening.

Often, a stroke leads to physical impairments such as hemiplegia or hemiparesis: weakness or paralysis on one side of the body. These impairments increase the risk of falling after a stroke. Therefore, a customized post-stroke exercise regimen should be created to help improve safety and independence.

Stroke prevention is another reason why exercise after stroke is important. Stroke is usually not an isolated incident, and risk factors often precede the stroke – such as high blood pressure, high cholesterol, diabetes, and obesity. Fortunately, all of these conditions can be improved with exercise.

While exercise is necessary for good health and recovery after stroke, it's important for patients to avoid over exercising. Pushing the body too hard can potentially result in regression or exacerbate conditions like post-stroke fatigue. Stroke patients will see the best results with a balanced regimen created with the help of a therapist. To get an idea of which exercises your medical team may recommend, let's look at the latest guidelines.

Guidelines for Exercise After Stroke

The best exercises after stroke depend upon your unique ability levels and pre-existing medical conditions. Many patients receive recommendations that prioritize stroke *rehabilitation* and stroke *prevention*.

Here are the current best practices as recommended by the American Hearty Association:

• **Gait training exercises** should be a top priority to help patients get back to "pre-stroke" levels of activity as soon as possible. Gait training can help improve independence with the Activities of Daily Living and improve tolerance for prolonged physical activity. Gait training is something that your physical therapist will need to help you with.

• **Aerobic exercise** should also be prioritized to help prevent another stroke. Experts recommend aerobic exercise after stroke for 20-60 minutes per day, 3-7 days per week. Dosage should be adjusted based on the patient's level of fitness.

• **Strength-training exercise** is recommended to reverse muscle atrophy, which typically occurs during the hospital stay and days thereafter. Strength-training programs should include light weights that allow at least one set of 10-15 repetitions. Strength-training should be performed 2-3 days per week with 8-10 exercises involving major muscle groups.

• **Stretching and range-of-motion exercises** are recommended to help improve flexibility and prevent contractures (a progressed condition of extremely stiff, tight muscles after stroke).

• **Balance exercises and core exercises** are recommended for patients at risk of falling.

It's important to work with your medical team to set your post-stroke exercise goals. For instance, some patients may need to prioritize gait training to develop the motivation for consistent aerobic exercise. Other patients with mild secondary effects might be able to accommodate both gait training and other forms of aerobic exercise.

No matter what your doctor or therapist recommends, one thing remains true throughout the stroke recovery process: **consistency and repetition matter**.

Why Repetition Matters

Some therapists refer to rehabilitation exercises as **neuromuscular training**, which focuses on training the nerves and muscles to communicate. After a stroke disrupts the pathways between the brain and muscles (resulting in impaired movement patterns), neuromuscular training can help restore movement by activating neuroplasticity. Neuroplasticity is the brain's natural ability to reorganize itself and learn new skills. This is how stroke patients can recover lost abilities like walking, dressing, and moving about your daily life. When discussing the best exercises after stroke with your therapist, you may hear them refer to something called massed practice. This refers to a large number of repetition used to stimulate neuroplasticity. The brain requires intense repetition to learn new skills because it likes to be efficient. When something is done frequently, it lets the brain know that task is important, and the brain responds by making that task easier to accomplish. Many therapists emphasize massed practice to help encourage as much neuroplasticity as possible.

Getting Ready for Exercise After Stroke

It's important for stroke patients to work with their healthcare providers to develop an exercise plan that accommodates their unique side effects and fitness levels. Doctors and therapists will likely encourage a unique combination of aerobic exercises to help prevent another stroke along with neuromuscular training to help recovery.

Stroke Support

There are many parts of stroke recovery where you'll need support of family or friends. During your hospital stay there are many questions that should be asked and that you should make sure that you understand the answers. According to the Heart and Stroke Foundation here are some of the questions to ask:

  • What type of stroke did I have? Was it caused by a blood clot or by bleeding into the brain?
  • What part of my brain is affected? What functions have been impacted by the stroke?
  • What will my recovery be like? What treatments will I receive? Will I need medication?
  • What are the results of my tests? What do they mean?
  • Did I receive a clot-busting drug?
  • Did the stroke affect my ability to swallow? Will I need a special diet?
  • What are my risk factors for another stroke? (this is especially important if you had a transient ischemic attack or mini-stroke.)
  • What is the next step in my care? Will I be admitted to hospital or discharged home?
  • Will I need rehabilitation? What types of rehabilitation will I be given? How much?
  • Will I be given an appointment at a stroke clinic or with a stroke specialist when I leave the hospital?
  • What will I be able to do in the next few months?
  • What can I expect one year from now?
  • What skills do my family and I need to take care of me? Who will show us how to do this?
  • What services and resources can help me and my family? How do I access them?

If you are a family member or friend of someone who's had a stroke, you might be wondering what the future holds. Some people make a full recovery and go back to their usual activities within a short time. But many others will live with the effects of a stroke for many months or years, and some effects last a lifetime.

You don't have to be living with someone to give help and support. You don't have to be there in person either; just showing someone you are thinking of them can help them feel that they haven't been forgotten. You could send a regular message, or make a phone call to share your news and ask how they are. Remember that rehabilitation and recovery can be incredibly difficult and hard work. They may be attempting to relearn some fundamental skills such as walking or talking, and this is a big challenge. You can help by giving encouragement and taking an interest.

Many people might not think of themselves as care givers, but simply as family members or friends helping out. You don't have to live with someone to be their care giver. You can take them grocery shopping, to the hairdresser or out to lunch. But it could also mean a daily phone call or emotional support.

How do you care for a family member or friend after a stroke? Tips for helping someone who had a stroke:

- Learn More About Stroke
- Don't Do Everything
- Encourage Rehab Exercises
- Understand the Invisible Side of Stroke
- Overcome Communication Barriers
- Provide Emotional Support
- Maintain Social Connections

Support

According to the Heart & Stroke Foundation, stroke is a sudden and life-altering event that may require an extended recovery period. It may result in new challenges in management of day-to-day limitations. Stroke can also have an impact on those close to you as your family and caregivers often take on additional roles. The healthcare team should be aware of this and ensure the proper support is available and that your needs are met.

After your stroke, you should be screened for level of coping, risk for depression, and other physical and psychological issues at each transition point. If issues are identified and the healthcare team receives your consent, you should be referred to appropriate services to address the issues and promote optimal outcomes.

Support is essential after stroke. You should be provided with information about peer support groups in the community where available and a list of community resources, including how to access these services, that will support your self-management at each care setting.

Tips for a successful recovery

Share your concerns. Your healthcare team should work with you to answer all your questions, help you identify and address your physical, emotional, mental and cognitive needs and provide education. This should happen at any stage or setting in your journey.

Write about it. Keep a journal so you can monitor your achievements and progress, record information about your medications or therapy, keep track of medical appointments, and write down questions to ask at your appointments.

Use a checklist. It can help you start a conversation about important issues you may be experiencing. Fill out a new one before every medical appointment. It gives you an ongoing record of your progress and makes it easier for your doctor, nurses or others on your healthcare team to understand how you are doing and work with you to get additional help if you need it. Add items that are unique to your recovery.

It's a team effort. Transitions of care requires the participation of you, your family and caregivers, health professionals and the broader community. It should involve collaborative goal setting, shared decision making and an individual recovery plan that is developed together and regularly reviewed and updated as you progress.

The power of community. If you have experienced stroke or heart condition, or are caring for someone who has, connecting with other people who know what you are going through can help the recovery journey. These communities share experiences, quality information and tips, while offering social and emotional support in a safe, inclusive and respectful community.

Medical Expenses

Depending on where you live, you can claim medical care expenses that are not covered by health plans. There is a limit to the amount you can claim. Keep all medical receipts and claim them at tax time. Expenses related to medical care that may be tax deductible include:

- Payments to medical practitioners, testing facilities and hospitals
- Transportation expenses
- Medical devices and equipment such as wheelchairs or orthotics
- Premiums paid to a private health insurance plan
- Expenses for adapting your home to your disability
- Costs of rehabilitation therapy
- Preventive, diagnostic and other treatments
- Medications
- Dental costs
- Alternative or complementary treatments

The Timeline for Stroke Recovery is Unpredictable!

The truth is that the stroke recovery timeline is unpredictable. How long it takes to recover from a stroke depends on many different factors, such as the size and location of the stroke, as well as your age and overall health prior to the stroke. The speed of treatment also has an effect on recovery outlook.

Some patients may recover completely within weeks of a stroke; others may take months or even years to fully recover; and still others may experience moderate to severe side effects on a permanent basis. You've got to keep positive, take your medication, work VERY hard, eat well, don't drink and don't smoke to get your best results!

Chapter 9
I Have Some Lessons That I'd Love to Share with You!

Having a stroke has changed how I look at life, how I feel about life and how I live my life!

Quite frankly, I never thought that having a stroke would be part of my life. Strokes were for people who either had family histories of strokes or cardiac problems, or people that lived unhealthy lives. On my maternal and paternal families there was no history of strokes or cardiac problems. I lived quite a healthy lifestyle. I didn't smoke; I quit 25 years ago. I didn't drink; I quit 12 years ago. I wasn't overweight. I exercised almost every day. I walked 10 kms/day and I love to play golf. But I found out that even when you do everything right, something can go wrong. "Stroke can happen to anyone, anywhere, anytime." says Dr. Kara Sands from the Mayo Clinic.

I have some lessons that I've love to share with you!

Live a healthy life! Even if it doesn't save you from a stroke, it will make it much easier to recover. I assure you that the fact that I walked 10 kms/day and worked out every day before my stroke, made it that much easier to get back into shape.

You have no idea how wonderful your friends are until you need them! I couldn't believe how wonderful my friends were during my stroke and recovery. Our relationships have really changed – for the better!

Support team! We all have friends that will support us. Have a list of their names and contact information. Have a friend set up a group on WhatsApp, or a similar type of service. That way anytime someone comes to see you they can sent out a text and anyone from around the world can read about it. My friends loved the WhatsApp group that my best friend Sue set up!

Ask for help when you need it! I lived alone so I needed help. If anyone offered to do anything for me I said, "YES PLEASE." Don't sit by, be a hero and say, "No, it's not necessary." You need help so take it when it's offered. I would never have walked 10 kms/day again if Judy K. hadn't come to my house and took me out walking. We started off slowly, but in four months I was back to 10 kms/day. In all honesty, I walked every day because I was driven, but take your time and you'll get there. My friend Sue took me grocery shopping once a week. I needed to buy food that I could microwave. You've got to eat!

Buy insurance! I know that when I say insurance that you think of medical/dental or travel insurance. But no, I'm talking about **Critical Illness Insurance** – covers you from heart attack, cancer and stroke, and **Independent Living Insurance** – covers you if you need help with two basic functions of living. I bought those two policies when I was 40, along with medical/dental and travel. Believe me, I wasn't so smart, but my friend Jane was in the insurance business and she sat me down and read me the riot act! And she was smart enough to tell me that if I didn't buy it at 40 that I probably wouldn't qualify later on because if you are on ANY drugs, you get refused! And the prices would be prohibitive! Critical Illness Insurance is the MOST IMPORTANT insurance. If you have a heart attack, cancer or a stroke you get a lump sum. You determine when you buy the policy how much that lump sum will be. Independent Living Insurance pays out if you need help with two basic functions of life. They pay you monthly and you determine how much your monthly payments will be when you buy the policy. I had my stroke at age 64 – no pension! If I didn't have my Critical Illness Insurance, I don't know what I would have done! It supported me for one year until I could apply for my pension. So please, apply for Critical Illness Insurance and Independent Living Insurance! Or at the very least – Critical Illness Insurance.

Give someone Power of Attorney and the ability to use your bank account! What would happen if you had a stroke and you needed someone to pay your bills and no one had Power of Attorney or the ability to use your bank account? Get your life set up properly! Make sure you give someone in your family or your best friend Power of Attorney and the ability to use your bank account. I gave it to my best friend Sue. Don't wait until you're in the hospital and have to scramble.

Make a will! I didn't have a will when I had my stroke, and my stroke was life threatening! I made a will as soon as I got home from rehab. But what would have happened if I had died????

Display medications, health conditions and your health care number! If you have a stroke and are taken to the hospital unconsciousness, someone needs to be able to find this information. I have mine stuck on the fridge.

Stay positive! After I recovered from my stroke all of my friends told me that they're sure that I recovered because I was so positive. I never walked around saying, "Poor me. Why me?". I woke up every day knowing that I had work to do and went ahead and did it. And, I had a smile on one half of my face (my face was paralyzed).

Take Charge!!!
When I was in the hospital nurses would come into my room and talk to who ever was in the room – but not me. I couldn't talk but I understood everything. My friends wouldn't answer them. They told the nurses to talk to me, and they did. Take charge!

Take charge and advocate for yourself! When you're in rehab as an inpatient or an outpatient, you can tell them that you want more therapy than they're giving you. When I was an inpatient, I had three hours of therapy, five days a week and physical therapy six days a week. I asked them for more therapy and I got an extra hour daily. And in that hour was a half hour with an electrical stimulus machine. So, I had four hours of therapy daily, five days a week and physical therapy six days a week. It was wonderful! Take charge!

When I was an outpatient, I also asked for more therapy, so my occupational therapist and physical therapist did a one-hour program that I could do at home every morning. I never missed a day! I'm convinced that I completely recovered because of all of the therapy that I got! Take charge!

Adjust your sense of style. I always wore very high heels because I'm five feet, 0 inches. No more high heels for me. After learning to walk again and having balance problems for the first year, I realized that I'd have to take lessons on how to walk in high heels. I gave them all away. Get over the fact that you're going to wear flats now and plan your wardrobe accordingly. If the worst thing that happens to you after you've had a stroke is that you have to wear flats, YEAH!!!!!!!!!!!

Talk, talk, talk! I know that you've had aphasia. So did I. But if you don't talk, you never will. Just go for it and when you've said the wrong thing, just laugh about it, like Sue and I used to do. We said "Jamaica" when I said the wrong word and laughed. Get rid of your insecurities and get out there and **TALK!**

Try new things and don't shy away if you don't do them well in the beginning! I joined pickleball. The first night that I went out **I did not hit a single ball!** Instead of slinking away and never going again, I started practicing in the garage until I started hitting balls. I went back the next time and I was better and every time I kept getting better. I **LOVE** pickleball! You can do it with anything that you put your mind to as long as you put yourself out there and **TRY**.

Try to make yourself look great! Get a haircut that doesn't need to be managed. As soon as you can, wear makeup! Four months after I had my stroke I was back to MAC's Russian Red lipstick, mascara and blush. My face was still paralyzed, but I could get my lipstick on. I always wore costume jewelry – big and gaudy!! I looked as close to myself as possible.

Try some of these things and please let me know if they work for you. They sure did for me!

Chapter 10
Normal Activities for Normal People

While you're recovering from your stroke, it's important to live your life as normal as possible. A few months before I had my stroke, I bought a piano. I live in an apartment building so it was an electric piano. And of course I bought headphones so I wouldn't get evicted. For years I kept saying that I really wanted to learn how to play but I never had the time or the space. It turns out that the electric piano fits perfectly in my entrance hall, and of course we always find the time to do the things that we really want.

I went to the Remenyi House of Music where they have all of the books to teach yourself or for a piano teacher to teach you how to play piano. It's a wonderful store! The books are all downstairs and on the main floor they have beautiful pianos and a host of other instruments. I spoke to one of the staff and told him that I couldn't read a note, so I wouldn't care if he gave me children's books but I didn't want to play "Twinkle, Twinkle Little Star." He assured me that he had adult books and sold me two books – Adult Piano Adventures Books 1 & 2. I went home and started. I just loved it! Then I had my stroke and for five months after that my right arm and hand were paralyzed. Once it started moving again, it took me quite a while to get my hand back to where I could attempt to play. So, I decided to hire a piano teacher. Lucky for me, there's a chap in my building who's a magnificent musician. He used to live across the hall from me and I was lucky enough to hear him play. Sadly he moved upstairs, but he was still in the building. I asked Scott if he'd teach me to play piano – knowing full well that what ever I had done before the stroke was GONE! Scott said yes! And so we began delightful piano lessons once a week.

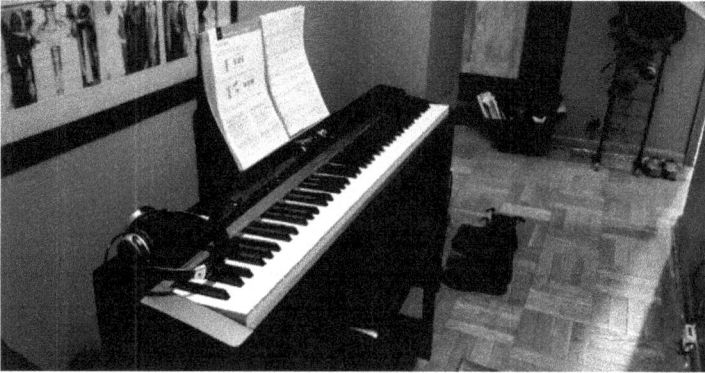

My Piano.

We started at the beginning. I had no clue about what I had done before my stroke. My right hand was still weak, but it could depress the keys, so I was learning how to play piano!

Golf Lessons

I LOVE! LOVE! LOVE! to play golf! I'm not very good. I started quite late in life. I gave myself golf lessons for my 50th birthday. I shoot between 105 -110 on an average day. On a great day I shoot between 95 – 99. On a disastrous day I don't keep score.

My right arm was still very weak, so I decided to take lessons. The first teacher that I had, didn't do anything for me. I told her about my stroke and how week my right arm was, but after a few lessons I moved onto another teacher. Mike was helping me make progress, but in reality I really thought that I just needed to get my right arm strong again. Boy, was I wrong!!!!

I had no idea that my brain wasn't talking to my right arm and hand. Your brain has to relearn many basic things, like how to operate certain parts of your body. But interestingly, Mike was teaching a guy to play with one arm because he'd had a stroke. Mike asked me if I could talk to him. I said, "Of course." He looked a little younger that me and after his stroke he couldn't use his arm at all anymore and he limped very badly. He wanted to talk about our strokes.

He wanted to know what hospital I was treated at and where I went for rehab. I told him that I was at St. Mike's and for rehab I was at Bridgepoint. He wanted to know about the rehab that I had at Bridgepoint. I told him that five times a week I had one hour of occupational therapy, one hour of physical therapy, one hour with the assistant occupational therapist and one hour of speech therapy, and six times a week I had physical therapy. After inpatient therapy I had outpatient therapy twice a week for three months. I asked him what hospital and rehab he was at.

He was at the North York General Hospital and for rehab he was at the Toronto Rehab. I asked about the rehab that he had. He told me that **TWICE A WEEK** he had one hour of occupational therapy, one hour of physical therapy and one hour of speech therapy. He didn't have outpatient therapy.

Oh my God, If I had only had therapies twice a week, I can't imagine the shape that I'd be in today! I feel so bad for him! And I feel so lucky that I had all the help I needed to work myself back to being me. I don't know why there isn't a strategy for all patients in all facilities to get the kind of care that I had. I don't know how many people are like this man who **COULDN'T** get better because they didn't have the resources. I want people to know that there are facilities who can give you exactly what you need to make a full recovery. If you land up in a place that gives you therapy twice a week, **DEMAND** that you change to a facility that will give you therapy six times a week and then give you outpatient therapy for three months.

I can only say that I was so incredibly LUCKY that I landed up at St. Mike's. Believe me, in a coma I had no idea where I was going to. But the EMS people knew that I had a stroke and they took me to the

Stroke Capital of Canada. And St. Mike's released me to Bridgepoint for me rehabilitation. I had the **BEST** and the **BEST!**

Sue and John and I went out golfing a few times. My right arm and hand were still very weak, but I had some fun hitting a few balls.

Chapter 11
My Gold and Platinum Awards

Sue

It amazes me even now to have Geri back, 99% the way she was before. Occasionally she will use a different word than before, but this is minor and no-one, but I would notice. Our shared experience has brought us closer and with a sense of deep gratitude that she defied the odds and recovered so well. It does change your perspective when you have a health scare and you realize how important your loved ones are.

Geri

Sue and I were best friends for close to 30 years and I always thought that we were as close as two friends could be. We met in Montreal, where we were both living. We were both avid tennis players and we played three times per week at an indoor club – Cote de Liesse Racquet Club. The club had a round robin with 32 participants, and that's how Sue and I met. We soon found out that we had lots in common from fashion to work to where we lived and we loved food. Becoming best friends just grew. After several years, Sue's company moved her to Toronto. The political situation in Quebec was really getting to me, so I accepted a one-year contract in Calgary.

Sue got a great condo rental because when a company moves you, they have to provide you with similar accommodations at the same price. This was an absolute joke because in Montreal the rents were dirt cheap. Sue and I were both living in three-bedroom flats for less than a one-bedroom flat was going for in Toronto. She was very lonely in Toronto and Calgary just wasn't for me. Sue kept calling and asking me to move to Toronto. I could stay with her until I found a place. Quite frankly, I was delighted at the thought of leaving Calgary, and I missed Sue, so I bought a one-way ticket to Toronto. It was a great move for both of us. I lived with Sue until I found an apartment, that I still live in today! Our best friendship saw us through Sue's marriage, the birth of her son, divorce and marriage to her fabulous husband John. Mine was a little different. I never wanted to get married or have children but our best friendship saw us through a variety of weird men and business contracts (I did corporate communications and change management for banks and insurance companies), some of which were fabulous and others that were nightmares. We really thought that we were the best friends that friends could be. This was true until I had my stroke.

Sue became a friend that you can't even imagine – better than a twin sister! I also want you to know that her husband John told Sue to spend what ever time she wanted to or needed to, with me. He would take care of her son Thomas. In case you don't believe that John is fabulous, let me tell you that he and Sue got married **ONE MONTH** before my stroke. He was and still is FABULOUS! Sue was in the hospital every day. She came to almost all of my tests with me. Sue became me – talking. We did everything together and believe it or not, we had fun! Even though I could only say, Yes, No, and Fuck, Sue understood everything that I wanted to say but couldn't.

When I was in rehab, Sue became my family. She did everything a family member would do. I gave her Power of Attorney and access to my bank accounts so she could pay my bills. Sue came almost every day and started taking me out for walks to the coffee shop. It was wonderful! She got my cheque from my Critical Illness policy and deposited it for me. Before I was released there was a "family meeting." Sue was my family.

Sue continued to do everything above and beyond the call of duty. She took me to the hairdresser, grocery shopping every week, out for lunch and I was invited to her house and she came to visit at mine. Sue came with me to my MPP, Jill Andrew, to get my driver's license back and then came for my first drive when I got it back. We went to St.

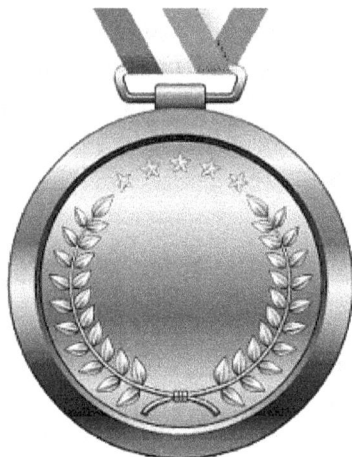

Sue Foster, My Champion.
My Platinum Medal goes to Sue. I could never have done it without her!

Anne's Spa for a weekend vacation, which Sue organized when we found out that I couldn't travel for a year. There was nothing that Sue wouldn't or couldn't do. So what ever I thought about our friendship before the stroke, it was nothing compared to what it became afterward. I will never have the words to describe how I feel for Sue, what she means to me and how eternally grateful I am for helping me get back to being me – but better!

One loyal friend is worth ten thousand relatives. Euripides

I have two Gold Medals to give out to my doctors – Dr. Daniel Selchen at St. Mike's Hospital and Dr. Heather MacNeill at Bridgepoint Rehab. I found out from Sue at the family meeting that my stroke was so bad that only one in four patients survive well. Dr. Selchen was one of the doctors at St. Mike's who gave me the clot-busting procedure. Even after I was released from rehab and I saw him for a visit, his secretary continued to call me up to one and a half years later to see how I was doing.

Dr. Heather MacNeill was my doctor from October 2018 – June 2019, while I was in inpatient rehab at Bridgepoint and she continued to be my doctor while I was in outpatient rehab. And she continued to see me for four months after that! I'm eternally grateful for the medical care and understanding that she gave me! Thank you from the bottom of my heart!

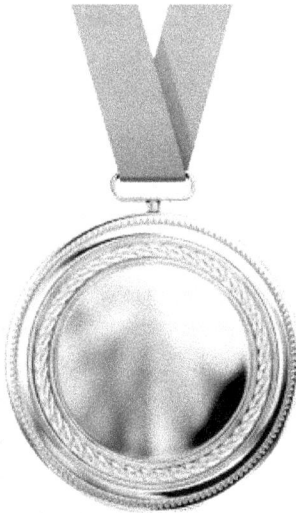

Dr. Daniel Seichen & Heather MacNeill.

Chapter 12
My 65th Birthday

I knew that I promised Shirley that I would have a 65th birthday party, even though I didn't like birthday parties. I kept thinking about what I should do when it finally occurred to me to make the party at the Toronto Wedding Chapel. My close friend Katherine owns the Toronto Wedding Chapel and she plans the best parties. I decided that I wanted to give a "thank you party" to my closest friends who did the most for me during my stroke. I invited Katherine & Everton (Katherine's husband), Sue, Pam, Sonya, Judy K. and of course Shirley. I made it very clear that there was not to be any cards or gifts of any sort! We were having a dinner party and it was Daeco Sushi who would do the catering. Aside from the fact and it's Sue's and my favourite restaurant, it is Shirley's as well. Every week I go and pick up dinner for me and Shirley (and sometimes twice a week). As soon as she finishes dinner, she tells me to tell the chef that this was his absolute best! My birthday is June 9th but there were some conflicts with the date, so we scheduled it for June 14th.

Janice couldn't come into Toronto for my birthday party so a few days before my 65th birthday Janice came into to Toronto. It was also really important for Janice to see Shirley. They'd been very close. We had a wonderful visit! Shirley loved to see Janice! We sat around talking and laughing!

Two Friends

Janice

I was so excited to see Geri for her 65th Birthday and since I am not big on driving on the 401, I took the train from Kingston to Toronto for the day. The train is lovely and much more my speed. LOL.

Geri was able to meet me at Union Station. We went for a coffee and had some girl time shopping, looking for some fabulous deals. I think I found some sandals that day. We had lunch with Sue who came to meet us at the Eaton's Centre.

I also REALLY wanted to see Shirley as her birthday was also within the same week. I just had this need to see her (sometimes you know things that you don't know). I am so happy that I had that opportunity to give her a hug and just spend some time with her. We had a great visit and I headed back home the same day. It was a day packed full of fun, love and friendship.

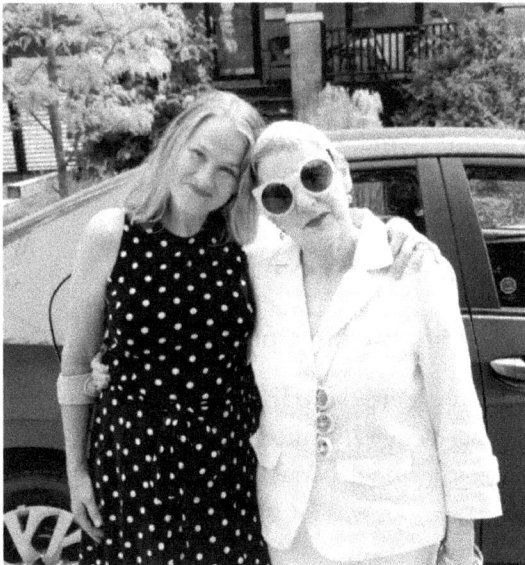

Sue and Me on June 9, 2019.
My 65th Birthday.

Geri

Sue and I went out on my actual birthday. That's my car in the background. I got my license back in May, so I was driving. YEAH!

I don't know even how to tell you this, but neither Sue nor I remember what we did on my birthday, or where we were going. Sue said that we must have been going somewhere nice because she was wearing her blue polka dot dress and had her makeup on. I always have my makeup on and I wasn't wearing anything special. Sue thinks that we must have gone to the Holt Renfrew Café or La Societe, but she doesn't remember. We talked and talked and talked about it, but NO, we can't remember. This is just like an episode that we had 25 years ago, that we still laugh about. It was a rainy, cold day in November and we got into the car and went out to the shopping centre. When we got there, we couldn't remember what we went for. We decided that we must have gone to the grocery store to pick up something, because why else would we have gone out? We walked up and down the aisles looking for something, but we didn't buy anything. Then we walked around in the shopping centre and ZERO – didn't buy anything. So we came home, sat down and watched golf on television. And we still laugh about it. Now, what we did on my birthday will take first place on the things that we forgot!

June 14 was my 65th birthday party and it is one to remember!

I picked up Sue and Pam (who lives in my building) and they came with Shirley and me. When I walked into the Wedding Chapel, it took my breath away! Katherine decorated the chapel in red – my favourite! Everything about the room was GORGEOUS! It was called for 6:00pm and everyone was there.

This was the first time that everyone was together and it was wonderous! And Shirley was the centre of attention! Katherine made Shirley beautiful black bibs (and she made her some to take home too). The sushi from Daeco Sushi was FABULOUS and everyone – especially Shirley – loved it!

Katherine

Being in the wedding and event planning industry we always needed new content written for our website and blogs. I always looked forward to meeting with Geri over sushi or rides to see vendors. Any opportunity to see Geri was welcomed.

As June would approach, I would ask Geri every year if she would like to have a party for her birthday and I would get the same answer, "No, let's just go for lunch." I would continue to try to convince her. "You love the Chapel let's just do it there." I had no luck but I did enjoy our annual birthday lunches.

After Geri's recovery I received an unexpected phone call from Geri. "I have been thinking I would like to have a thank you / birthday party. Would the Chapel be available?" Those words were music to my ears. With much excitement we were off to planning the long-anticipated party. I met with Geri to discuss the details of the party. It was so important to Shirley that Geri was celebrated not only for her birthday but for her incredible recovery. Nothing but celebrations all around! I was just thrilled!

As we begin planning Geri's party the invitations were sent. The theme was red because that's Geri's favourite colour. We purchased the red lantern. We ordered the sushi. The day had arrived and the look on Geri's face was worth the 20 plus years of waiting for the "party." Shirley's reaction once she arrived at the venue was of joy and happiness and fulfillment.

The joy to be a part of this wonderful day is evident on each guest's face. We were so thrilled that we were chosen to host Geri's celebration to thank all her friends for their input in her spectacular recovery - grocery shopping, laundry, walking daily to restore her mobility, or just a simple phone call to say hello. We all knew that Geri's recovery was vital, and she had chosen us to be part of her journey.

Geri, thank you for your tenacity, your persistence and love for life, your friendship, great sushi lunches and your fabulous taste in jewelry!

You have taught us so much. The great life lesson you have taught me is never to give up. All goals are achievable no matter how unachievable they may seem at the time. May you continue to walk with strength, talk with courage and know that you are forever surrounded with love.

Pam

It was almost surreal that here we all were, really just a short time later, celebrating Geri's birthday - with her walking and talking and back to her wonderful self. It was such a privilege to spend that time with Geri and all her friends and, most especially, her mom, Shirley. This was far more than a birthday party, it was a celebration of life and thanksgiving. You could feel the love and gratitude in the room, it was palpable. We shared stories of Geri and her friends and family, how each of us met her and I know that we were all so grateful that Shirley was part of this celebration – she was the heart of Geri's family and loved by all who met her.

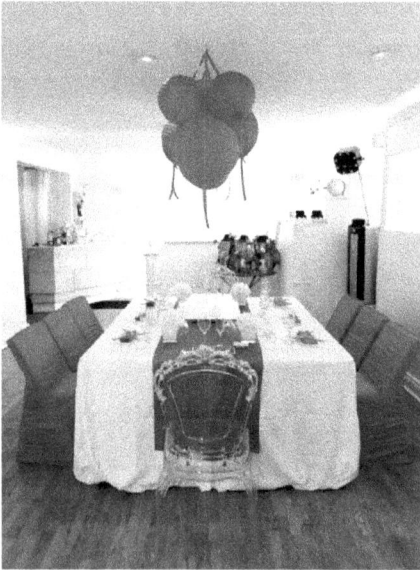

Katherine decorated the chaplel in red—my favorite.

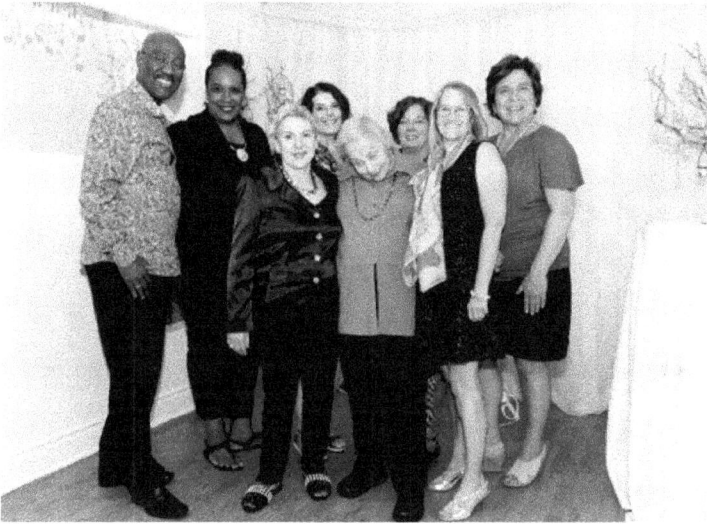

Everton, Katherine, Sonya, Pam, Judy K., Me, Shirley & Sue.

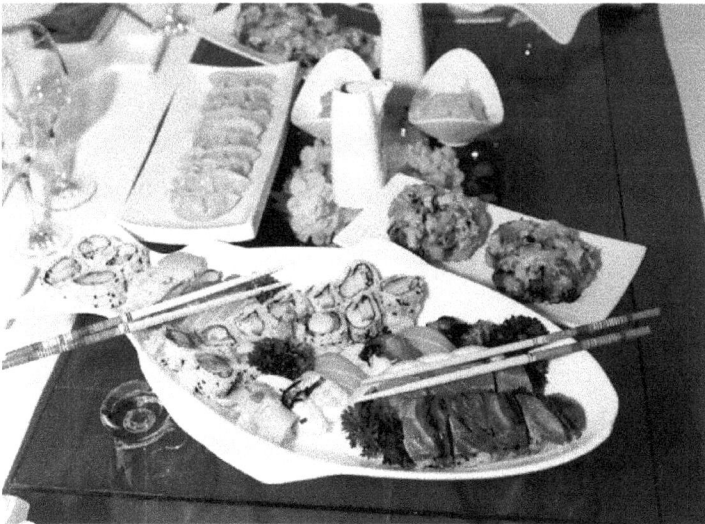

Fabulous Sushi!

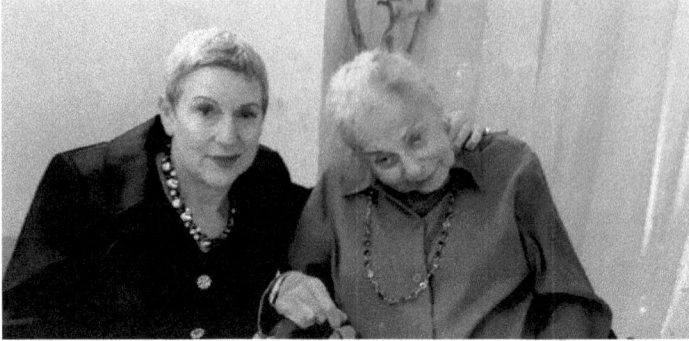

Me & Shirley.

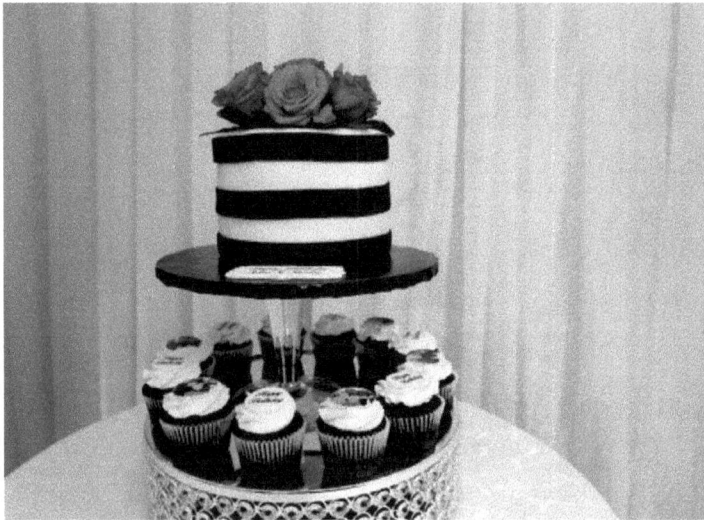

Fabulous birthday cake that says "Happy Birthday Geri & Shirley"
whose Birthday was June 18th &
"Amazing Cupcakes with My Pictures."

The party was fabulous! I gave a "thank you to my friends" speech. I meant it from the bottom of my heart! If not for **my mother** and these **six absolutely extraordinary friends,** I would not have lived, recovered, and I was continuing to recover. My face was still partially paralyzed, my right arm and hand were weak and although I was now walking 10 kms per day, I had no balance. But I had overcome the most difficult stuff in nine months.

The fabulous birthday cake was for me and Shirley (her birthday was on June 18). It was delicious as were the cupcakes with my pictures on them. Katherine thought of absolutely everything! I don't know how I could ever thank Katherine for everything she did while I was in the hospital and rehab and then recovering at home, and for making the **EXTRAORDINARY 65ᵀᴴ BIRTHDAY PARTY!**

It was getting late and Shirley was getting tired, but she had the most WONDERFUL time. As I drove us home, I get wondering what would happen now that Shirley had watched me recover from my stroke and she had just attended my 65ᵗʰ birthday party…

As June came to an end, I had my last appointment with Dr. MacNeill. It seemed fitting. I was driving my car again and I felt great! But, I would miss her. She looked at me and said that she didn't have anything to examine me for any more. We gave each other a hug and I walked out of her office. Her secretary came over to me and said, "Geri, I never want to see you here again!" And we both laughed.

I then went up to the third floor to see everyone that had taken care of me while I was an inpatient. It was a lovely visit.

Chapter 13

Shirley's Death

Sue and I were over at Shirley's one afternoon and Sue was telling Shirley about an Indian dinner that she and John had. Shirley got excited and said that she'd never gone out for Indian food, which amazed me because she and Joe had travelled all over the world and I thought had eaten every kind of food. We asked her if she'd like to go out for an Indian lunch and with a big smile on her face she said, "Of course." The next day, we set off to Sue's favourite place – Banjara's.

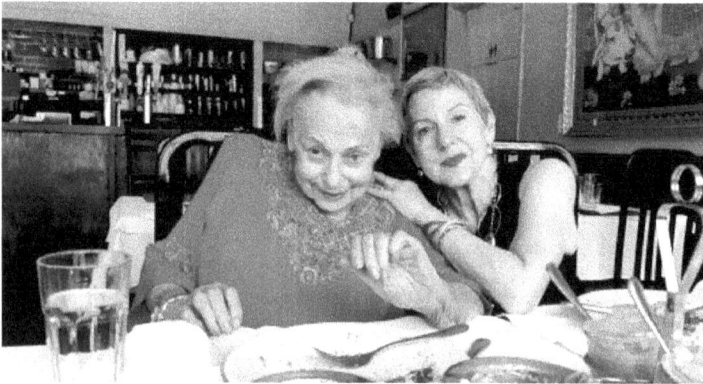

July 9, 2019.
Shirley & Me at Banjara.

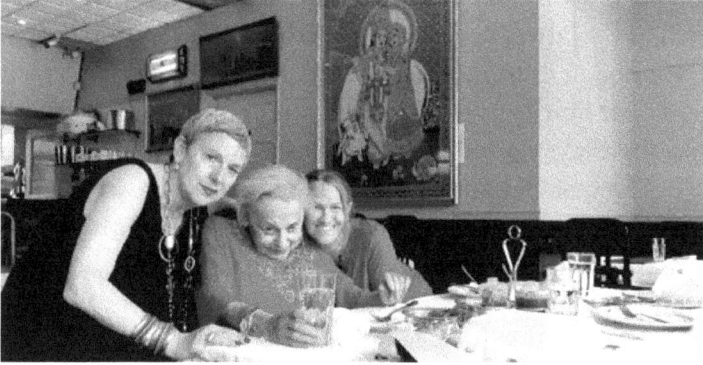

July 9, 2019.
Me, Shirley & Sue at Banjara.

Oh my God! Shirley loved Indian food! She ate with such gusto! And we were really lucky that the owner was there and he treated Shirley like a queen. It was fabulous!

Life was back to "her normal" for Shirley. One day, August 6, 2019, her nurse told me that he thought that Shirley had an infection in her leg. Sue came with Shirley and I as we set off to Mount Sinai Hospital

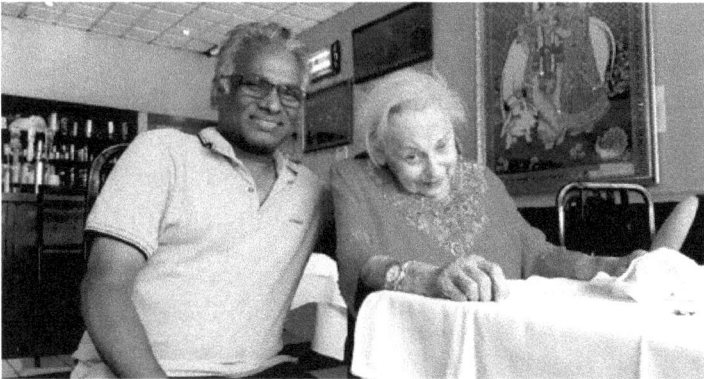

July 9, 2019.
The owner of Banjara & Shirley.

on Wednesday, August 7, 2019. It's so much easier when Sue comes with us so I can leave Shirley with Sue at the hospital and go park the car.

We were waiting at Emergency until a doctor was ready to see Shirley. They've always been so wonderful to Shirley any time she was there. The doctor examined her and said, "Shirley, how are you today?" Sue leant over Shirley and told her to speak up so everyone could hear and that there was no mistaking what she wanted. She looked at him and said, "Doctor, I want to die." He looked at me as my eyes were filling up with tears. But, I wasn't surprised. When I thought back to the time that my father died and she told me that she wanted to die with him but that she was staying alive for me. She stayed alive and had saved my life. If Shirley had been dead, so would I. And in the last few months she kept telling me that she wanted to stay alive to see me recover from my stroke and to attend my 65th birthday party. She did both of those things and now she could go to be with my father, who had been waiting for the past six years.

The doctor admitted her to a very large room. It was big enough for my closest friends to come and visit. The doctor said he believed that she'd be dead by the morning (Thursday). I called Erica (her granddaughter) and Saundra (her daughter-in-law, Erica's mother) in Calgary and they would be arriving on Friday. The doctor removed all of her medication and told me that if she was twitchy to call the nurse and she'd give her a shot. Sue and I were staying in the hospital. I only had to go home to get my medication. Thursday morning Shirley was still with us, but slowly fading. Pam came every day and Katherine came every night. Hour by hour, she continued to fade. I kept telling her that I loved her. She heard the same from Sue, Pam and Katherine. Erica and Saundra arrived on Friday. Shirley was still alive – obviously waiting for Erica and Saundra to come and say good-bye. After that Shirley needed to hear that she had my permission to go and so I gave it to her. At 1:00am, Saturday morning, August 10, 2019, Shirley was gone.

Sue

I was determined to be part of Geri and Shirley's journey. My wonderful husband and supportive son understood and gave me their blessing. It was a sad but very beautiful time. I remember telling Shirley that I would be there for Geri. Shirley wasn't speaking at that point, but she gave my hand a lovely warm squeeze. After Erica and Saundra had visited, it became clear that Shirley was nearing the end of her journey. Geri with a broken heart, gave her permission to leave, and she peacefully took her last breath. I remember above all a strange and wonderful sense of peace in her room for the whole week.

Geri

I called the Jewish funeral parlour. We were going to bury Shirley on Sunday. Sue and I left the hospital around 2:00am. Sue went to her house and I went to mine. I cried and cried and cried... I didn't know that I had that much water in me, but this time I was crying for Shirley and Joe because when Joe died, I had to take care of Shirley. I stayed in her apartment with her for three weeks. I had to hold back all of my tears and take care of my mother. But this time I was taken over by tears! I had no one to take care of...

I took a shower and went up to Shirley's apartment. I cried and cried and cried... I called Erica and Saundra around 8:00am and they came over. They were going to leave that evening, so they wanted to help me go through Shirley's stuff. We went through Shirley's clothes and made the bags to give away. Shirley had beautiful art and crystal and china, so I asked Erica what she wanted. Erica chose Shirley's wedding china, a large, framed wedding photo, two paintings and a needlepoint. She took the wedding china and the wedding photo, and I shipped the two paintings and needlepoint to her. Erica and Saundra were a big help getting the clothes sorted out before they went home. I would deal with the rest.

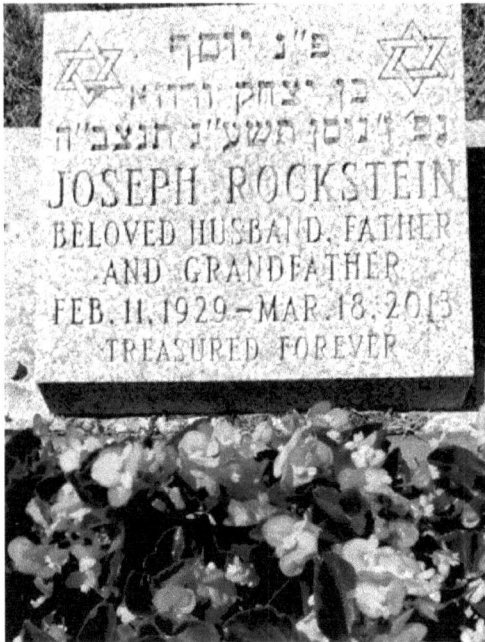

Joe's Marker.

Shirley was going to have to same funeral as my father's. Before Joe died, he told Shirley that she wanted his body to be given to science. Shirley almost had a heart attack. Then Joe said that he wanted to be cremated. Again, Shirley almost had a heart attack. Joe finally agreed to be buried in a Jewish cemetery, but it had to be the cheapest thing possible! And he didn't want a big stone, he wanted a stone marker. Shirley agreed and told him that she would have the same when she died. Here is the stone marker that we had made for Joe. Shirley will get the same.

Would Joe have approved that I ordered the flowers? Definitely NOT. He HATED all monies spent for funerals or at cemeteries! I ordered them for Shirley, so that when we went to the cemetery, Shirley saw flowers.

Two Friends

I gave Shirley the same funeral that I gave Joe. It was a graveside service. Sue, Pam and I were the only ones at the grave. Katherine was going to cancel her weddings (she owns the Toronto Wedding Chapel) and come, but I said absolutely NOT. Erica and Saundra left for home on Saturday evening. The Rabbi gave the service. It was over…

Sue, Pam and I went to the Centre Street Deli to pick up all kinds of delicious food to eat at Sue's place. We ate and talked about nothing but Shirley and Joe. And we laughed and cried.

Joe had waited six years for Shirley to join him. He visited Shirley every day in her apartment and was with me every morning at the hospital. Now they're together for eternity. Their love story was something so special, I often wonder if that's why I never married because I could never find anything that came close to what they had. They met at a B'nai B'rith dance when Shirley was 17 and Joe was 19 and fell madly in love! Two years later they walked down the aisle on October 29, 1950. They had a beautiful, extraordinary marriage that lasted 63 years, always in love. When ever you'd see them walking down the street, they were always holding hands. And they were loving parents to my brother David and me and wonderful grandparents to David's daughter Erica. They were always thinking of ways that made the family unit a wonderful thing. My friends always loved coming to our house because there was always laughter and joy. I still talk to Shirley and Joe every morning and I know that they can hear me. One day I'll be with them again.

Judy S.

Having grown up with Geri, I also grew up with Shirley and Joe. They were fantastic! Joe was never flustered by anything. Even when I had a car accident near their country house, instead of getting excited, he started cleaning snow off the windows while waiting for the police. "Just keeping busy"! He always had a smile, and loved his "goodies" that Shirley kept in steady supply. Shirley was the consummate mother hen. She loved to cook and bake, and it was always a joy to spend sleepovers at Geri's and be part of her family. They were a joyful, loving couple and that spread to include all around them.

Janice

In August when I received the phone call from Geri about Shirley's passing it was an extremely sad day. Shirley, like Joe was such an amazing person. She was beautiful inside and out! I remember the very first time I had Montreal Smoked meat with Shirley, Joe and Geri. You would have thought that there were 20 people in the room when there was only the 4 of us. The exuberance for life was amazing. The laughter and the conversation created an electric atmosphere to be in. I also remember that the smoked meat was incredible...I really ate way too much! Shirley and Joe loved it! I am laughing to myself just thinking about that day. Still fresh in my memory.

Pam

I didn't know Geri's dad, Joe, very well, I was fortunate to have met him a few times and loved him at first sight. He was just an amazing man and I knew he and Shirley had a real life-long love affair and he was such a proud father to Geri. Of course I was devastated for Geri and her mom when they lost Joe but Shirley's passing was, for me, so very difficult. I had the chance to really get to know Shirley. I helped her when I could when Geri was in Bridgepoint and we spent a lot of time talking. What mattered to Shirley was her family and though Joe had been gone a few years by then, to her he was still there. She thought of him every day and missed him terribly. Shirley's time now was for Geri and while hard to say, she looked forward to seeing Joe again soon. She just needed to know Geri had her life back. She already knew she had the support of her friends, especially Sue, and she was ready to go. Unfortunately, we, and especially Geri, were not ready to say goodbye. Shirley was a homemaker. Her life was her family and she was a true lady – with a fantastic sense of humour! Shirley only gave good to the world and I truly pray that she is rewarded for this by once more being where she wanted to be, with her Joe.

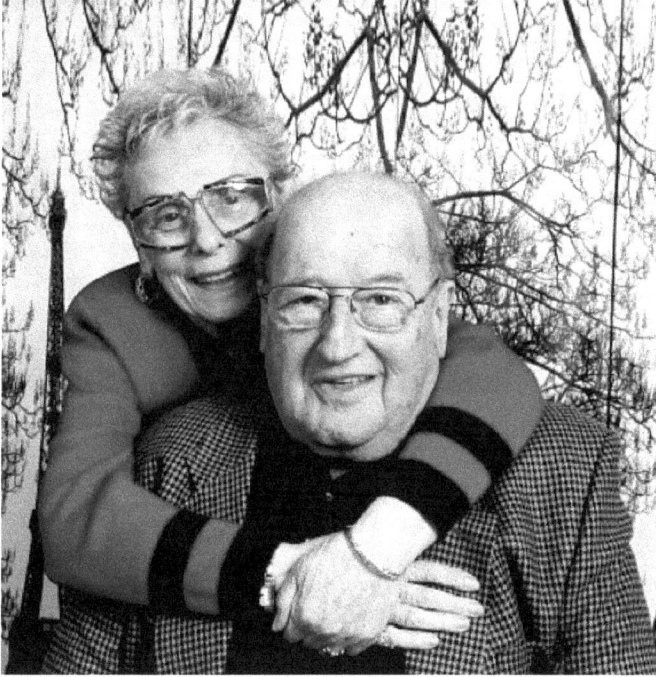

Shirley & Joe on Joe's 80th Birthday.

I still had Shirley's apartment to deal with. I invited my friends over to see who wanted any of her beautiful things. I had taken the things that I wanted. I was very grateful that all of the beautiful things were taken by my friends which would have made Shirley very happy. Then I invited her nurses and personal support workers in addition to people that lived in the building to come and take a few things. Everything was gone. I didn't sell one thing; I gave things to people who I knew would value them. I closed the door and gave back the keys. Again, it was over...

I was over at Sue's and her dog Kyser came to grieve with me. Kyser never lets me down.

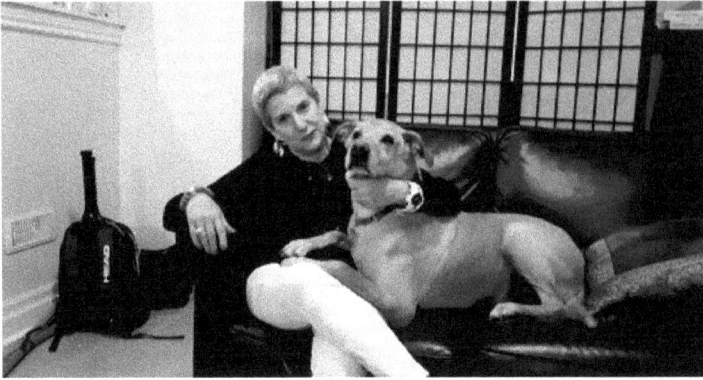

Me & Keyser Grieving.

A few days after Shirley's death, I was talking to Janice. She asked me to come to Kingston and visit. Janice said that I had nothing to stay in Toronto for anymore. I decided to go, and I had Shirley's crystal bowls and serving pieces for Janice. She entertains a lot, and it would make Shirley very happy that Janice was using them.

It did me the world of good to be with Janice and the family. I cried when I had to, but we laughed and Janice and I did the things we always did – we shopped and talked. We went to our favourite shop in Newboro – Kilborn's and we got some amazing sales. And then we went on to Picton. It was wonderful. We had a wonderful lunch and enjoyed all of the stores. I felt normal! The weekend did me the world of good!

Janice

Geri came to see me the next weekend after Shirley passed away. It was a very difficult time for her and still is. I am honored that she wanted to come and be with me. All I could do is give her a hug and be there for her. We talked about Shirley and Joe and enjoyed the beautiful dishes that Geri brought for me that belonged to Shirley. I have one of the glass cutting boards on my counter beside my stove as it works extremely well as a spoon rest for me. What a beautiful love story that Shirley and Joe had. What terrific parents Geri was blessed with! It's hard to look at the pictures and not tear up but the memories of them make you smile.

Chapter 14

I'm Starting
to Live a Normal Life

My friend Jane called at towards the end of August and asked if Sue and I could come to her office (Desjardins Insurance) and give a talk on how I recovered from my stroke. They were having a fund raiser for the Heart & Stroke Foundation (who had written an article about me and Sue that was published in July) on September 4, 2019. Sue and I said yes! We worked really hard on a PowerPoint exhibit to be the background for our talk which would run about 30 minutes. We had two of my neighbours, Joan and Don, to come into my apartment so that we could try it out. We did, made a few changes and we were ready.

September 4, 2019, we drove to Hamilton (where's Jane's office is) for lunch and then to give our talk. There were about 50 people in the audience. Sue and I really enjoyed it. The audience was really into it and asked many questions to which we had answers. We got a huge round of applause. Afterward the director wanted to know if we were on the tour (paid to speak)!

I've been wanting to go back to yoga for some time. I wanted to get my balance back and rebuild the strength on my right side. Unfortunately, the only yoga in my neighbourhood was a hot yoga studio (I was given a free class) and when I walked in it was like a hot steam bath, so I walked out and never did the class. I was drenched! The only other yoga was in Good Life. I was a member of Good Life for six months when they bought my gym, so I did yoga there and

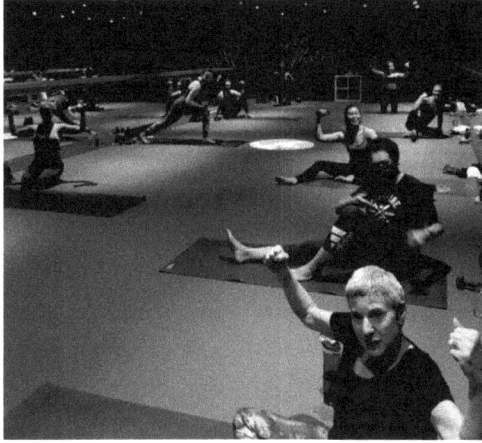

Yoga class. I'm in the front right.
It was at the beginning because I had no weights.

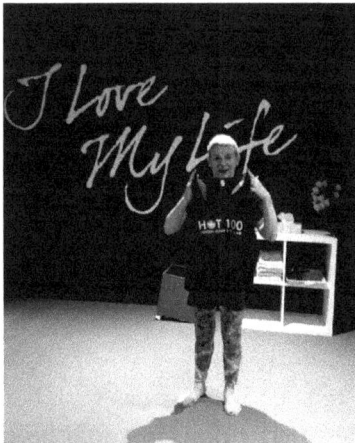

I hit 100 classes! I got the t-shirt as a gift, but I didn't put it on
becasue I couldn't wear it.

really didn't like it. I left Good Life, who was buying every gym in Toronto.

I was walking in my neighbourhood one day when I saw men putting up a sign that said, "Oxygen Yoga Fitness." There was a man watching what they were doing. He told me his name was Daniel, that he and his wife owned it and that they would be open on November 4, 2019. He gave me literature about it and it looked just like the place that I would love! I went back the last week of October and signed up. This studio is also hot yoga, but it's dry heat – 38 degrees. It's wonderful! I met his wife Ronit who would be running the studio. Ronit and Daniel Wilk are absolutely WONDERFUL! Because of who they are, they hired the VERY BEST instructors and run the studio in the VERY BEST way. I told them about my stroke and that I was still recovering. I still had no balance, and my right arm and hand were very weak. They said that it was no problem. Yoga is for everyone. I spoke to each of the instructors before taking a class so that they would know. I got a mat space near the door in case I had to get out for a break and when I started. I used to step out about three times per class. I couldn't use weights because of my right side, but it really wasn't a problem. I had no balance. I couldn't even pick up one foot, but there was lots of progress to be made. There were things that I couldn't do, things that I struggled to do and a few things that I could do. But I kept going and each day it got a little easier. I started going to yoga 6 – 7 times per week and I was getting stronger and getting my balance back. I loved going to yoga and still do go 6 mornings per week! I take off Thursdays because I go grocery shopping in the morning and I don't like to do an class in the afternoon.

Christmas at Janice's

Janice invited me to spend Christmas with her, Len, Ty, Ryker, Mac the cat and Rosco the wonder dog. It would be a wonderful break!

There wasn't much snow, so I drove down to Kingston for my four-day visit. I was so excited to see Janice and the family! Janice's decorations are beautiful, as you can see by the photos.

Janice and I did "girl's stuff." We went to our favourite shops all around the town and some out of town. The girls had ground to cover.

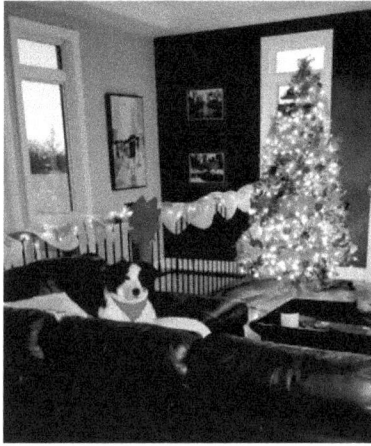

Christmas 2019.
Rosco & the beautiful decorations!

But, I made sure to help Janice make a wonderful Christmas dinner! And we had plenty of food for lunches afterward.

I went home four days later, sad to say good-bye, but I had the VERY BEST time!

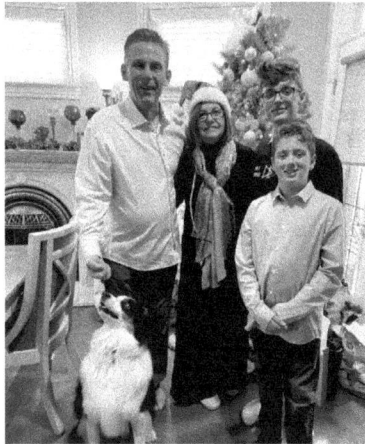

Christmas 2019.
Rosco, Len, Janice, Ty & Ryker.

Chapter 15

Bad News & Good News
& Bad News

My friend Judy S.'s daughter Marla was getting married on January 25, 2020 in Montreal and I was going! I'm Auntie Geri to Marla and I love her to pieces! Marla lives in Toronto and she came to visit me regularly. I took the train in because you never know how the weather is going to be. And I booked at a Best Western Hotel on Peel and Sherbrooke. It's convenient for walking around downtown.

Unfortunately, my old friend Lise was dying of ovarian cancer. Lise and I have been friends for 40 years. We lived next door in the same apartment building for 17 years. She was diagnosed with stage four ovarian cancer five years before. After chemotherapy and radiation, she was great for two years, but then her cancer came back. They did more chemotherapy but couldn't do radiation because the cancer had spread. Then chemotherapy didn't work any more, so she started on drug trials. Now five years later I was basically going to say good-bye.

I've been calling Lise every day just to say hello and let her know that I was thinking about her. She told me that I could come to see her, but the maximum that I could stay was one half hour. And there was a possibility that she would ask me to leave before that. Lise couldn't have people stay very long. She had to lie down. I told her that I didn't care if I stayed for one minute, but I wanted to come to see her. I knew that it would be the last time.

The wedding was the evening of Saturday, January 25, 2020, so I made arrangements to go to Lise's apartment at 10:00am. I arrived promptly at 10:00am and when Lise opened the door we hugged and hugged and hugged. Lise had plenty of makeup on and she'd lost a lot of weight, but she was still beautiful!

We just started talking like the old days, and before I knew it, it was 1:00pm. I didn't stay for one half hour, I stayed for three hours! Lise was very frail and tired, so I got up to leave. The good-bye was one of the hardest things that I've had to do! This is Lise on January 25, 2020.

I walked back to my hotel, window shopping along the way, but I couldn't shake the mood. I cried most of the way. I stopped to get a pastry and coffee and continued walking. I had to change my mood. I was going to see one of my oldest friends, Judy S. and her daughter Marla, who was getting married.

I was wearing a fabulous, beaded dress — it was totally beaded - and sequined booties! I landed up with sequined booties because I found out that since I had my stroke, I could no longer wear heels, but I could wear booties because the heels are wide enough to give me balance. I assume that learning how to walk again, my right leg being weak for so long and my balance was still not perfect, were all contributing

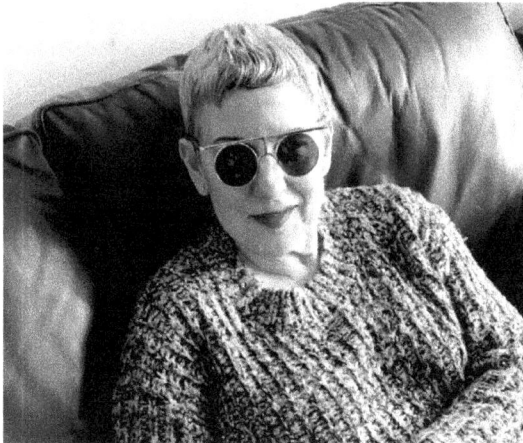

I was visiting Lise.

factors. If all I had to pay for recovering from my stroke was no high heels, I was happy to pay! While I was in Nordstrom's they had sequined booties. I tried on the booties and I was in love! I bought them instantly. So I brought a beaded dress and sequined booties to wear to the wedding!

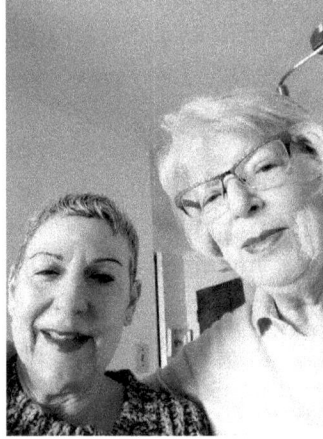

Me & Lise in a selfie.

I took a taxi to the wedding and I had arrived. When I walked in the first person that I saw was Sandra, Judy's other daughter, and also my niece. We had a great, big hug!!!! And then I saw Judy! It was the first time that I'd seen her since she came to see me in rehab. Oh my God, did we hug and kiss!

Judy S.

No guest was more important to me that day than Geri. Knowing her miraculous stroke journey, and that she travelled from Toronto to get here, made her presence extra special to me. She's watched my girls grow up, and they call her Auntie Geri. She looked fantastic, and she was perfect, and she was Geri! Everyone in my family and many of my friends know her, so she had many people to catch up with and I was thrilled that she was there.

The wedding was beautiful, and Marla and Adam were spectacular! It was wonderful to see so many people that I've know since I was a teenager and in my 20s. I was shocked that so many young people came over to me and said, "Great dress." I was incredibly flattered the entire evening.

I had great catch-up conversations with so many of Judy's friends and family. I sat with one group, then another and then another. Everyone knew about my stroke and they wanted to hear how I had recovered. If they didn't know that I had had a stroke, no one would have known.

The clock struck 12 and everyone was leaving. One of Judy's friends offered me a ride to my hotel. We all said our good-byes, happily!

The next morning, I walked to the train station and headed home.

Now it was finally time to look for a job. I was working at Scotiabank when I had my stroke, but I was working on contract, so there would be no job waiting for me. After recovering from my stroke, I had Shirley to take care of. When she died, I really needed to recover. I got my resume in order and started looking. I was applying for contract work as I had for the last 30 years.

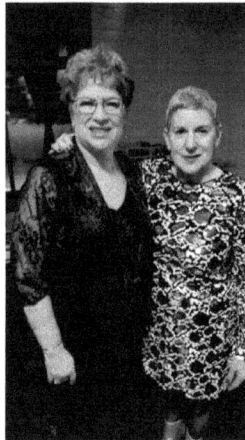

Judy & Me at the Wedding.

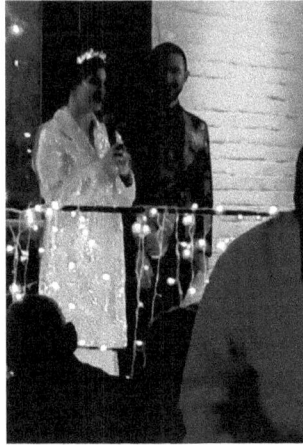

Maria & Adam are happily married.

So, I had a relatively normal life. February brought Sue's birthday. We went to Mezzetta Café & Restaurant, a fabulous Mediterranean restaurant! Sue and I have been going there for over 25 years. We found

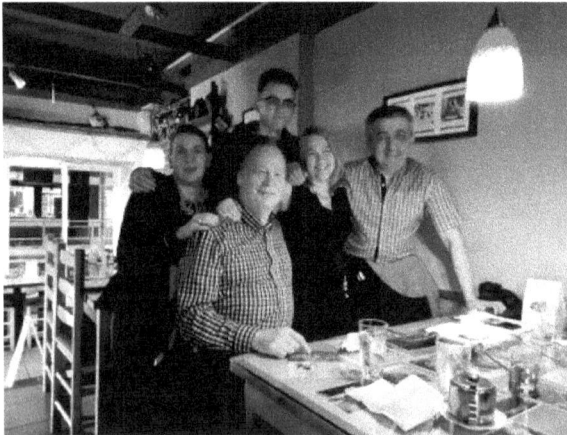

February 27, 2020.
John, Sue, Safa (the owner of Mezzetta Café & Restaurant)
Me & Thomas at Sue's birthday dinner.

it quite by accident. One evening we were out walking on St. Clair, going to an Italian restaurant that we both enjoyed. We were talking so much that we realized that we had already passed the restaurant, but we stopped in front of Mezzetta's. Sue knew that I loved Mediterranean food and so did she, so we went in. We met the owner, Safa, who is just marvellous! And from that night onward, we were regular customers!

In the beginning of March I telephoned Lise (as I did daily) and her sister answered. She had just taken Lise to the hospital. Lise had fallen. Later that day her nephew called me to say that Lise was dying and he would call me to let me know. That evening he called to say that Lise had died... I'm so eternally grateful that I had three hours with her in January!

COVID -19 descended upon the earth! In the blink of an eye my life and everyone's life changed dramatically!

Chapter 16
Living in a COVID World

I live alone and I'm a very social person, but I live alone, and now I have to be alone! I can't get together with friends except to go for a walk outside. Oh my God! This is an impossible way to live!

Sue and I started to go walking every day with Kyser. Kyser was already 10 years old, but boy was he getting exercise and in magnificent shape. John joined us on the weekends.

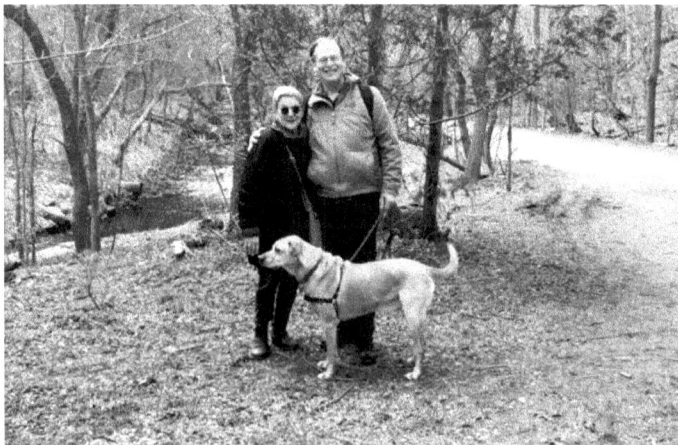

April 2020.
Sue took the picture of Me, John & Kyser in the revine.

No more piano lessons for me! My teacher wouldn't come to my apartment. I decided that I would continue on my own, rather than just wait until COVID calmed down. Who knows when that will happen!

My yoga studio (all gyms and studios) was now closed. I had to look for yoga classes on YouTube and find some that I liked. I was very lucky that one of my favourite yoga teachers at the studio, Danielle, said that she would give me a yoga class once a week via Skype on Sunday mornings. It was wonderful! I told her that I wanted to concentrate on my balance and opening up my hips. And, Danielle made it happen!

Looking for a job was now over for me! They weren't hiring anyone and if they want to hire a contractor, they'd hire someone young that they can pay a fraction of what they would have to pay me. So, I would have to file for my pension NOW! I really thought that I'd go back to work, but now, if I don't have my pension, I wouldn't be able to pay my rent.

All the stores are closed. When I go for my long morning walk, you can't even go in anywhere to have a look.

Restaurants are all closed, but they allowed them to open their patios and they could have heaters. Judy K. and I went out for brunches on Saturdays, so now we could continue to get together.

Pam and I started going out for walks after her work was done and sometime on the weekends. I've also started to come to terms with some things in my life. I found out that I did most of my driving because of Shirley. When I went grocery shopping for her she wanted "this from Superstore, this from Metro, this from Loblaws, this from Sunny…" And on the weekend I would love to take her out, but she liked to go to places we could only go to in the car. Shirley died last August. In October I put on my snow tires and I took them off in May. I went to Kingston twice and I had a grand total of 1,000 kms! It was time to get rid of the car. I've leased my cars, so someone referred me to Lease Busters. They were fabulous and I sold my lease within a week!

The golf courses were open, but they had very strict rules! There had to be 12 minutes between tee off groups. When you arrived you had to put on a mask to go in and pay – only one group at a time. I really wanted to try and get my right arm working again. It was still weaker than my left, but getting better. Golfing was WONDERFUL! We tried

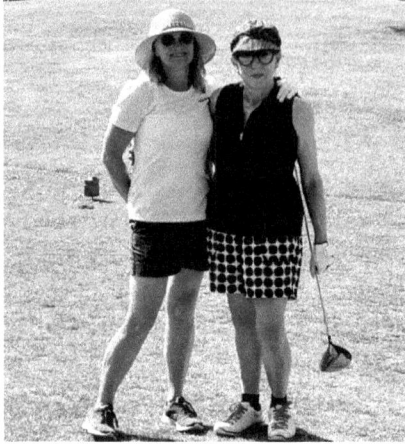

June 22, 2020.
Sue & I at Scarlett Woods. John took the photo.

to go every second Sunday. I was the one who booked the times because you could book five days in advance and the phones opened at 7:00am. This is clearly not a time for Sue! And John was getting ready for work. Sue and John kept score. I didn't. Maybe next summer when my right arm is strong again, I'll start keeping score. I'd give anything to shoot between 105 – 110 again! I was never a great golfer, but now that it's taken me so long to build up the strength in my right arm, I'm going to feel that I'm a super star when I can shoot 105 – 110!

Sue and I decided that we would help local businesses. Daeco Sushi was our first choice. We went there once a week for lunch and we never missed a week! The food was fabulous and we could eat on their patio.

Sue was getting ready to pursue her book business – MemorableLives.ca. And the book that she'd written about Shirley was ready. We were very lucky that Shirley had read the book and absolutely loved it before she died.

In July I took the train and went to Janice's. Kingston was much more open than Toronto. You could eat in restaurants and the stores were all open. But most of all I got to spend a weekend with Janice, Len and the kids and of course Rosco the wonder dog!

Two Friends

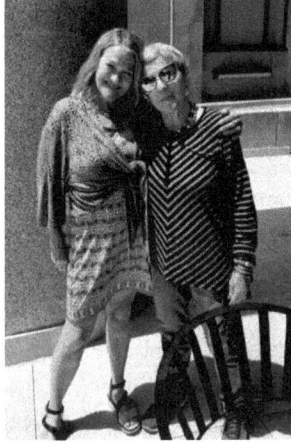

June 25, 2020.
Sue & I outside Daeco's—the best sushi in Toonto!

Their house is wonderful! They have a wonderful salt water pool out back and a fabulous barbeque. We swam, we ate and we had a terrific time. Of course Janice and I did "girls stuff" too! How could I come to Kingston and not shop?

The yoga studio opened again, with limited capacity on March 14, 2020. Yeah!!!! Danielle and I cancelled our Sunday sessions, and I took them in the studio.

The rest of the summer Sue and I continued walking around Toronto, looking for good places for coffee with patios. We found a really nice coffee shop that is unfortunately not there anymore.

My God, I can't believe it! It's two years since I've had my stroke! Judy K. and Sue took me out to lunch to celebrate. Restaurants with outdoor patios were still open.

* * *

It feels almost like it wasn't me who had the stroke. I can't remember what it felt like to wake up and have my right arm, hand and leg paralyzed. I can't remember what it felt like not to be able to talk and only to say Yes, No, or Fuck. I can't remember what it felt like to lie in a bed and to make in my diapers for an entire month! I can't remember what it felt like to be tube fed for an entire month. I can't remember all of the speech therapy, occupational therapy and physical therapy that I had at Bridgepoint and for three months there as an outpatient. I can't remember how terrified I felt when I saw stairs. I can't remember how scared I was when Judy K. came to take me out for our first walk. I can't remember how petrified I was to go out walking on my own. I can't remember how it felt not to be able to wear my red lipstick because half of my face was paralyzed. I can't remember how scared I was to come home from rehab and to have to do things for myself. I can't remember how terrified I was to take a shower on my own. I can't remember how I overcame all of these things, but I did, and I slowly but surely put my life together again. I'VE RECOVERED 100%. Thank you to my friends who have made it all possible! I'm wearing my red lipstick again. I have the complete use of my right arm and hand and leg. I'm not afraid of stairs. I'm walking 10 kms per day and doing yoga every day. I talk way too much!

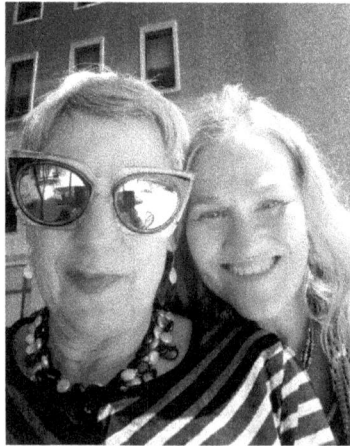

June 22, 2020.
Our selfie!

Two Friends

Sue

Two years later on, there are parts of Geri's journey that remain imprinted in my brain, while much else has faded with time. We will never forget what happened, but it is not front and centre of our worlds anymore. And yes, some things haven't changed, Geri does talk too much! But I wouldn't have her any other way.

Judy S.

Geri is my hero! She is the poster child for strength of character, fortitude, and perseverance. She is focused and energetic, and strong-willed. These are the traits of a champion. Because of her competitive nature, she made it a mission to conquer her adversity, and do it well. If anyone could beat this, it was Geri!

She is a chameleon, who has reinvented herself many times, in many places. I have known her and loved her through all her incarnations. And I am the better person for having been there on her journey.

Geri is a people magnet. She has been able to accumulate good friends wherever she set herself down. I am thankful that I am one of the longer-standing ones, and am grateful to the "new" crew who supported her through these last 2 years. She has named you all, but I want to add my gratitude to you for taking care of my friend Geri while I was far away. In distance only......

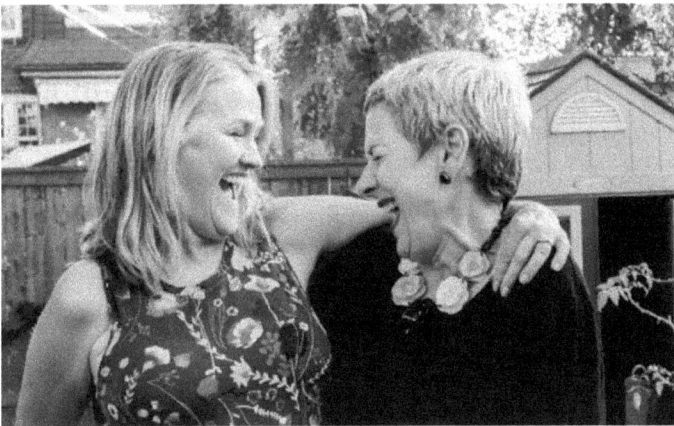

September 8, 2020.
Sue & Me in her backyard.

Becoming a Volunteer

Once it finally sunk into my head that I wasn't going to go back to work, I had to find a place to volunteer. I'd been volunteering my whole life. For 40 years I had been volunteering with Special Olympics and just loved it! I head coached a swim team. Long ago in a galaxy far, far away, I was a competitive swimmer. But now, I wanted to give something back to stroke patients. I didn't know where to start so I sent an email to Ryan, my speech therapist at Bridgepoint. He suggested that I give my time to the Aphasia Institute. Quite honestly, I didn't even know that there was an Aphasia Institute.

What is Aphasia? Aphasia is a condition that robs you of the ability to communicate. It can affect your ability to speak, write and understand language, both verbal and written. Aphasia can be extremely stressful for both the individual who had the stroke and their family and friends. Speech is such a significant part of human interaction, and it's something that most people take for granted.

According to the Aphasia Institute, aphasia is a communication problem that **masks a person's inherent competence.** It is usually the lasting result of a stroke or brain injury, but may also be caused by other neurological conditions such as dementia or brain tumours. Aphasia is not well known or understood and may be classified as an 'invisible' disability.

People with aphasia have a language problem. This means that talking and understanding including the ability to communicate opinions, feelings, thoughts and emotions is hard. This has a devastating impact on human connection – the ability to interact and have conversations with people. Without the ability to **participate in conversation**, every relationship, every life role and almost every life activity is at risk. **Conversation is core to the ability to participate in virtually every realm of adult life.** The result is often loss of self-esteem and profound social isolation. Reading and writing are often also affected which makes aphasia even more challenging.

BUT

People with aphasia do know what is going on. Even when the aphasia is severe, many are capable of participating in decisions that pertain to them if the appropriate support is provided – similar to giving a wheelchair or walker to someone who can't walk. The abilities of people with aphasia are often underestimated when there is a problem with understanding what others say. The easiest way to grasp this is to think of yourself in a country where you do not speak the language. You would not be able to express yourself, understand others, read or write – but this does not mean that you would not know what you want to say or communicate.

All People with Aphasia:

- Are still intelligent
- Know what they want
- Are competent adults
- Can make their own decisions

Symptoms

Aphasia is a symptom of some other condition, such as a stroke or a brain tumor.

A person with aphasia may:

- May not speak at all
- Speak in short or incomplete sentences
- Speak in sentences that don't make sense
- Substitute one word for another or one sound for another
- Speak unrecognizable words
- Have difficulty finding words
- Not understand other people's conversation
- Not understand what they read
- Write sentences that don't make sense

Patterns of aphasia

People with aphasia may have different strengths and weaknesses in their speech patterns. Different aspects of language are in different parts of the left side of the brain. So your type of aphasia depends on how your stroke affects parts of your brain. According to the American Stroke Association:

Wernicke's Aphasia (receptive)
If you have Wernicke's Aphasia, you may:

- Say many words that don't make sense
- Use the wrong words; for instance, you might call a fork a "gleeble"
- String together a series of meaningless words that sound like a sentence but don't make sense

Broca's Aphasia (expressive)
Injury to the frontal regions of the left hemisphere impacts how words are strung together to form complete sentences. This can lead to Broca's Aphasia, which is characterized by:

- Difficulty forming complete sentences
- Leaving out words like "is" or "the"
- Saying something that doesn't resemble a sentence
- Trouble understanding sentences
- Making mistakes in following directions like "left, right, under and after"
- Using a word that's close to what you intend, but not the exact word; for example, saying "car" when you mean "truck"

Global Aphasia
A stroke that affects an extensive portion of your front and back regions of the left hemisphere may result in Global Aphasia. You may have difficulty:

- Understanding words and sentences
- Forming words and sentences

These patterns describe how well the person can understand what others say. They also describe how easy it is for the person to speak or to correctly repeat what someone else says.

Can you fully recover from aphasia? According to the Mayo Clinic few people regain pre-injury communication levels. I am one of the **VERY LUCKY** few who have regained my pre-injury communication levels!

Family and friends can help. Some people mistakenly think those with aphasia aren't as smart as they used to be. They certainly are! But they can think; they just can't say what they think. So please if you're talking to someone with aphasia, PLEASE treat them as you would any competent adult. You can help people with aphasia express themselves by:

- Asking yes/no questions
- Ask one question at a time
- Write keywords down
- Paraphrasing periodically during conversation
- Modifying the length and complexity of conversations
- Using gestures to emphasize important points
- Establishing a topic before beginning a conversation

I followed up on Ryan's recommendation to contact The Aphasia Institute. It was founded in 1979 by Pat Arato (1938-2020). It's a Canadian community-based centre of excellence with an international reputation as a world leader and educator in aphasia. They train people how to work with members to overcome the communication barriers aphasia creates and help them re-engage in everyday life based. It's based on training that they've developed at the Aphasia Institute – Supported Conversation for Adults with Aphasia (SCA).

It sounded perfect for me. I applied to be a volunteer and after an interview, I was accepted. Yeah!

Continuing Living With COVID

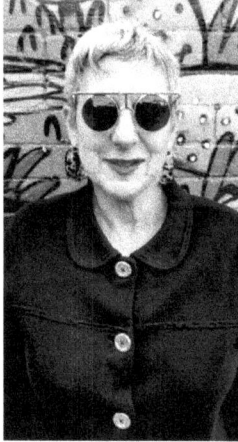

October 2020.
Judy and I had lunch on our usual Saturday and then we
went walking through Graffiti Alley. Look at the colours!

Unfortunately, the yoga studio was closed again October 10, 2020. But Ronit and Daniel really gave it some thought and they reopened virtually and they were going to keep it opened this way! It was fabulous! We had the same teachers giving the same classes. There were not as many classes as when the studio was live and in person, but it's just great!

Thanksgiving 2020 was upon us and we could still travel within Ontario. I booked the train and went to Janice's in Kingston. It was wonderful!

Janice is a fabulous cook. I was the sous chef! We cooked, we ate and of course we did some shopping.

Janice and I took Rosco out on walk down by the water. It was cold!

In November Toronto was locked down – no restaurant patios, no stores, no nothing!!! And I couldn't go to Kingston anymore!

Two Friends

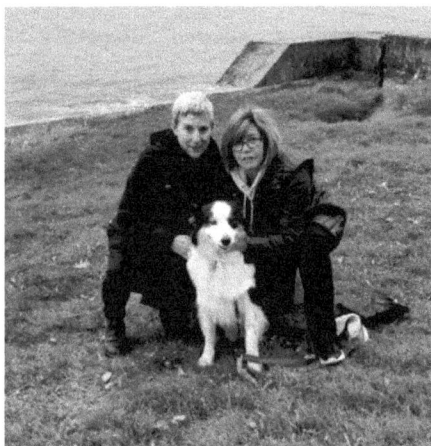

Me, Janice & Roscoe.

Chapter 17
My Modeling Assignment

I know a photographer, Natalia Dolan, who lives in my building. She's in her 30s and she's just lovely. On February 22, 2021 she sent me these texts:

"I may be doing a photoshoot Friday at my Studio. I have to confirm with my client today. It pays $250, for about an hour of your time, and you would just be with me and Dayna. We'd just need to be from a distance haha. But I'll only know confirmation later today!! And I'm not sure if you're even available then.

You would just be your funky fabulous self with any funky eye glasses if you had any. And you could keep all the shots for you to use on LinkedIn or your site."

You don't have to guess that I said YES! She got approval and we were scheduled for Friday, February 26, 2021. I asked her what she wanted me to wear and suggested that she come to my apartment and have a look. Nat showed up with her mask and chose my red jacket and my sunglasses.

On Friday I showed up at her studio. Her best friend Danya was there to help. I had so much fun. Nat took about 100 photos!

Here are several photos that were taken for an ad for *Indeed*.

This is how I went form a life-threatening stroke to a 66-year-old model! But, there's more!

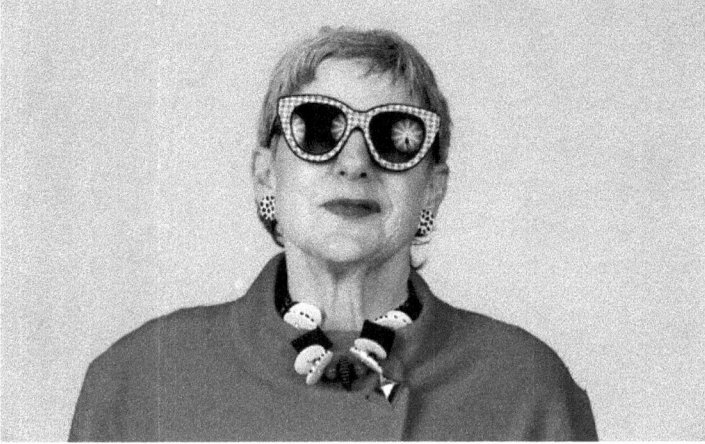

February 26, 2021.
My modeling assignment.

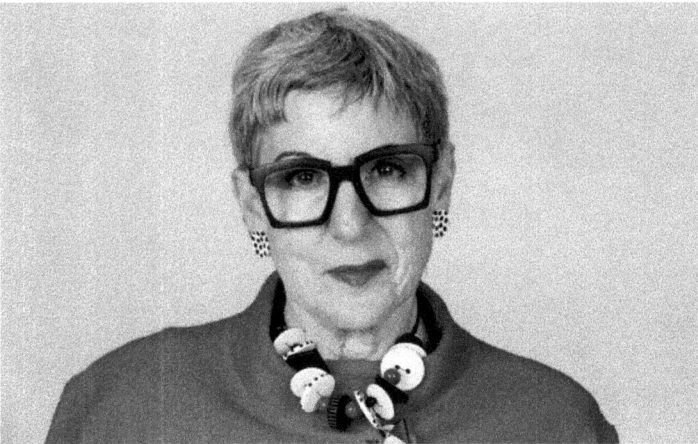

February 26, 2021.
My modeling assignment.

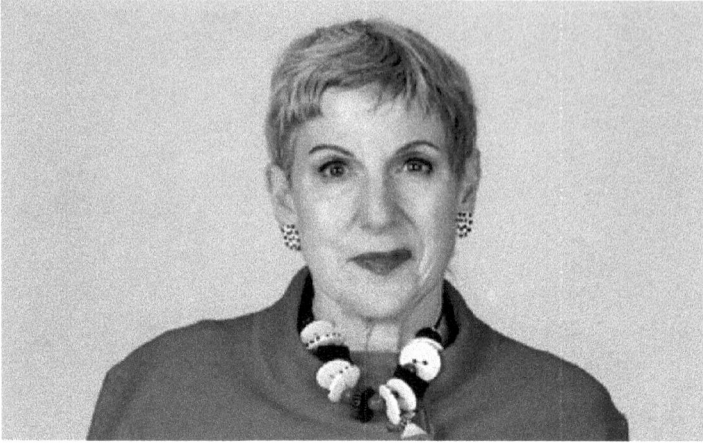

February 26, 2021.
My modeling assignment.

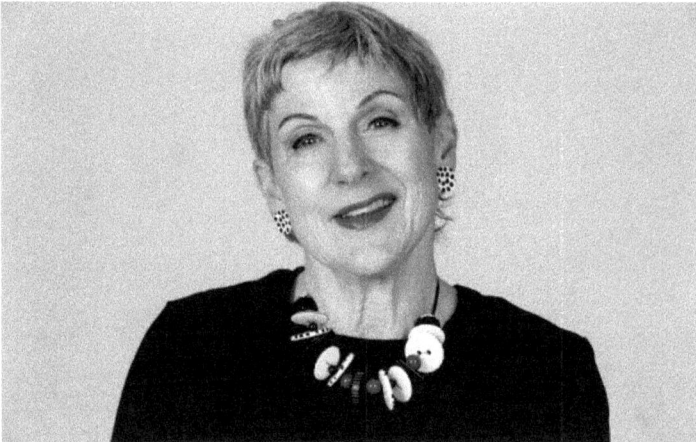

February 26, 2021.
My modeling assignment.

Chapter 18

Sue & I Become Cover Girls

I got a call from the editor of *Best Health Magazine* in August 2021. They were doing their October/November issue on **Good Company. Why Friendship is Vital to Your Wellbeing**. Nat Dolan, the photographer who did my photos for Indeed was as well doing the photos for Best Health Magazine. Nat knew the story of my stroke and how **ABSOLUTELY INCREDIBLE** Sue had been to me during my recovery and still is, so she told the editor our story. The editor loved it and asked if we could be featured in a article in their October/November issue. Sue and I said, "YES!!!".

We asked Nat what we should wear. Nat came down to my apartment and chose my red linen dress and my turquoise necklace. We then showed it to Sue and Sue chose her blue polka dot dress. A few days later we went to Nat's studio to have our makeup done and the writer of the article was there to listen to our story. I told the makeup artist that she could do anything she wanted except change my lipstick. I've been wearing MAC's Russian Red for probably 35 years and I still love it like no other shade. Sue and I changed clothes and had our makeup done, while telling our story. We had such a great time!

At the end of September, the magazines were delivered to my house. When I looked at them I almost fainted. Sue and I were on the cover!!!!!

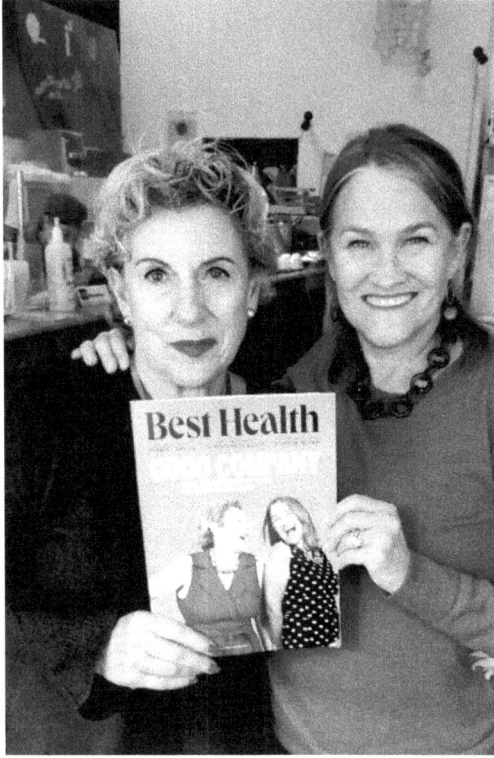

Me & Sue on the cover of *Best Health Magazine*!

So I wasn't just a model, but Sue and I were **Cover Girls**!!!

Chapter 19

My Brain is Playing Hard to Get

In the summer of 2022 Sue and I decided to back on our usual golf holiday in Northern Michigan to a resort call Boyne Highlands. It's a fabulous resort and we had been going for 11 years, until I had my stroke. I finally felt secure that my right arm was back to it's usual fine form so I called to make the reservations. Oh my God, it would have cost us double the price of when we went in 2017, so we couldn't go.

We had some really good friends and positively lovely people that we first met 11 years ago – Bob and Gail from Los Angeles. Our first year there, when we arrived at the resort there was a welcome party for the guests and Bob and Gail were the only ones who spoke to us. Everyone else thought we were a gay couple, because no women came without men. For all the years after that we arranged to be there at the same time. After a few years Bob and Gail bought a beautiful house on the property and in the last few years, Bob had semi retired so he went down in May and stayed until September. Gail came down every month because she was still working full time.

I sent Bob and email and told him that Sue and I couldn't come down because the prices were astronomical! Bob said, "Don't worry. Come stay with me." Sue and I were thrilled and we told Bob that we would do all of the cooking for the week. We went to the Boyne Highlands from June 10 – 17. En route we stopped to pick up some groceries and wine and when we pulled into Boyne Highlands, I started to cry. I never thought that I go back and golf!

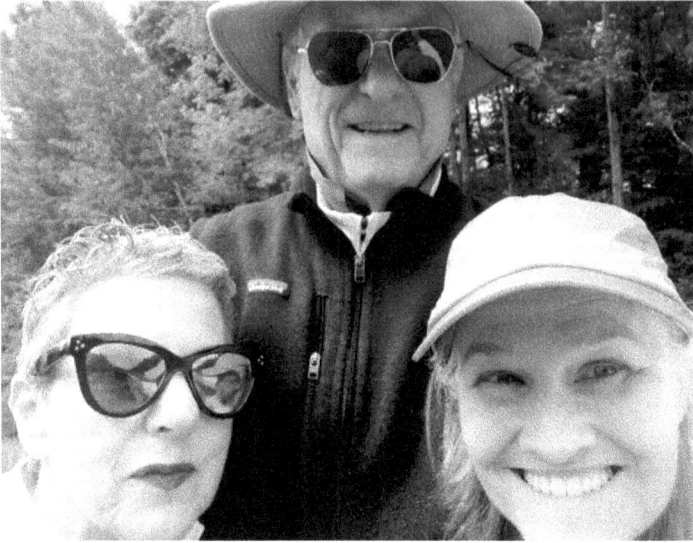

Me, Bob, & Sue.
Our selfie! Bob the Giant. Geri & Sue, Shrimps!

Unfortunately, Gail wasn't there that week and we missed her, but we were so happy to see to see Bob!! I made my Cousin Helen's meat loaf for dinner. Sue and I checked out what Bob had and didn't have. We made a list and we would go out shopping after golf the next day.

We booked our favourite courses – The Hills and The Heather! They are so gorgeous!

The courses were as magnificent as always. My right arm and hand were as strong as ever, but my golf game was missing. I knew exactly how to hit a shot, but my brain didn't send my arm and hand the message. It seems that my brain refused to communicate with my right arm and hand! I was shocked because I can do everything else with my right arm and hand – write, cut, sew, tweeze, cook and anything else that you can think of. Sue gave me a golf lesson as a birthday present (my birthday was June 9), but I discovered that it didn't do me any good because it didn't feel comfortable to me. We all have our own way of hitting. I finally realized that on the occasion when my muscle memory kicked in, I could drive 150 yards with my 5 wood – my favourite club. I didn't want to relearn how to play, but I could find my muscle memory.

I didn't golf very well – never kept score, but we had a SUPER week! And we saw some of our favourite people who work at Boyne – Josh Richter who has now become the Senior Vice President of Golf Operations. He invited us for lunch and we had a fabulous time catching up. What was very interesting was that one of the golf pros at Boyne had a stroke and Josh wanted to know how to help him. We had a very long chat about it and we saw him several times after that. And I was writing this book, so I sent it to Josh who used it to help his friend! I'm so delighted that it helped someone! And we saw Ray who is a Golf Marshall. Ray was now 80 years old and looks fabulous, but best of all he remembered us the minute that he saw us!

This year in the spring I'm going to keep going to a driving range, get a few buckets of balls and keep hitting them until my brain can recreate my muscle memory for every shot! I've finally discovered how to get my golf game back.

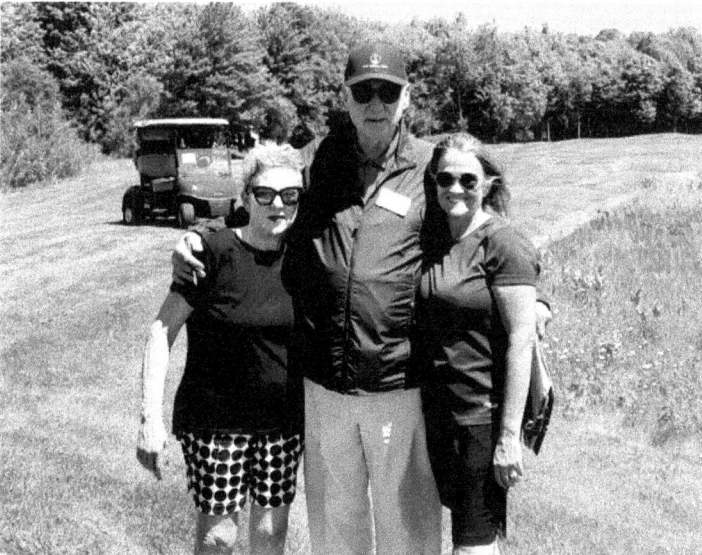

Me, Ray, & Sue.

I recently started playing pickleball. Sue's husband John was interested and Sue is an avid tennis player, so she had no time, but I told John that I would join him, although I had no idea about pickleball. You can find out about anything on YouTube!

It's winter so we're going to Brown's School and Community Centre on Tuesday and Thursday evening from 7:15 – 8:45. And this couldn't be more convenient for me because Brown's is about one block south of my apartment building on the same street! There are three pickleball courts set up in the gym, so that allows for 12 people playing at the same time. They cap it at 24 players. When one game is over, the people leave the court and another group comes on.

We arrived on the first Tuesday and I thought that I wouldn't have trouble with pickleball because I was a very good tennis player and a good athlete. Well, you guessed it! My brain wasn't telling my right arm and hand what to do. I couldn't hit a ball – **NOT ONE**! Everyone was really nice and didn't make me feel bad, but I apologized to everyone and came home and decided to practice in my garage.

I live in an apartment building with underground parking. I had to find a space where two cars, side by side, were out of the garage and I found one. So I said, "Hello Brain. Stop being so independent! You have to start talking to my right arm and hand because when I asked them why I couldn't hit a ball they said it was because you wouldn't tell them how to do it. This is enough of your bad behaviour. Let's all work together!"

Gradually I started striking the ball. Thursday, I was back at pickleball and I hit a few shots. Back to the garage, where I kept practicing. Tuesday came and I was better. On Thursday, my fellow pickleballers all said that I had a good serve and I was hitting the ball.

I'll keep going to the garage and keep practicing! Then we had a cold spell and practicing in the garage was not in the cards. But, strangely enough, I kept getting better – slowly.

On Thursday we were warming up close to the net. I could never hit a ball close to the net. Well this Thursday I rarely missed one. Then we started playing and I couldn't believe it! I was hitting balls and my brain was telling my arm and hand what to do and they were listening.

My fellow pickleballers were watching and cheering for me! I actually won two games that night and everyone was telling me how wonderful I did! And I'll keep reminding my brain that we're in this together – the brain, right arm and hand together - not separately. I could never have accomplished anything at pickleball if not for the wonderful group that I joined. If they hadn't been so nice and encouraging I would have never gone back after my first attempt. They are fantastic, especially John, Richard, Meg, Tommy and Amy! And Richard and Tommy give me playing tips!

Now, I think that as I keep getting better at pickleball, it means that my brain is communicating with my right arm and hand. I can feel it. In the beginning I just hit the ball. Where ever it went, I was happy as long as I touched it. After playing six times my brain decided where to hit the ball. My backhand had come back. Slowly I was developing a pickleball game. YEAH!!!

The interesting thing is that I started taking golf swings at home, and they felt really comfortable, which means that my muscle memory has kicked in and my brain and my right arm and hand are communicating. So pickleball may be the best thing to give me back my golf game. I just needed something to make my brain communicate with my right arm and hand!!!! Our brains are a wonderful thing! YEAH brain!!!

Chapter 20

Am I So Different Since the Stroke?

Am I so different since the stroke? **YES!!! Physically and emotionally!**

I actually look different because my hair is now curly. I've had sticks straight hair my whole life, but during COVID, the hairdressers were closed for nine months. As my salt and pepper hair got more salt, my hair got curly because of the "salt curls." I really liked it so I continued to wear it a little longer.

Before my stroke I had a very busy life. I was working full time at Scotiabank in Communications and Change Management. I worked out five days a week and did yoga on the weekends. And in the summer, I golfed. Pam and I were subscribed to the National Geographic series and Judy K. and I were subscribed to the Mirvish Off Broadway series. I had a membership with the ROM and the AGO. When I had any free time, I got together with friends. I took my mother grocery shopping and out on the weekends. I rarely had a free moment.

I rarely thought about how much I liked my friends. They existed and were part of my life. My life just went on.

But the biggest change in me is that I have great love for my friends! YES! LOVE! I can't forget everything that they did for me. And they did it voluntarily! No one asked them, but they gave of themselves – to me. I don't know how I was lucky enough to have

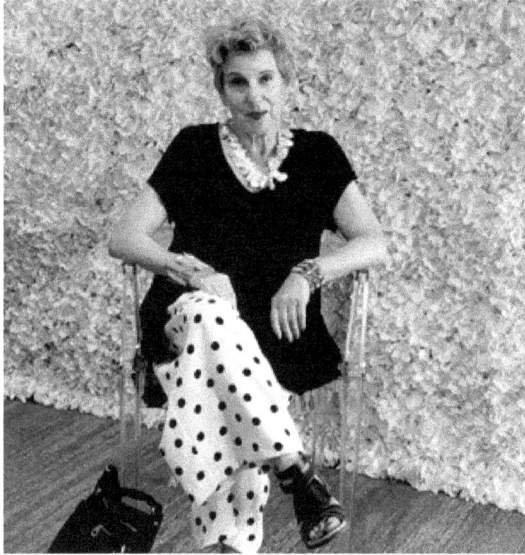

Me.

friends like this in my life, but I was, and still am. Every day when I wake up, I never forget how wonderful my friends were, and are! I can't believe that I never slowed down enough to recognize how wonderful my friends were and still are. I really missed **A LOT**!!! And I wonder how much else I missed!

I'm not as busy as I was before the stroke. Sue and I have an every morning check in and if one of us is missing we really do get nervous! The stroke keeps preying on our nerves, even though we won't admit it. Katherine continues to still check in on me every day. I still do a little work for old time clients and friends. I don't work out during the week and go to yoga on the weekends. Instead, I go to yoga six mornings a week. I love how yoga makes me feel. And it gave me back my balance and strengthened my right side. I have no interest in lifting weights and riding the bike. And I walk about 10 kms/day.

I'm getting back into sports. I love golf and my brain and hand are now communicating, so I know that I'll have a wonderful summer. And my newest love – pickleball! My group told me that in the summer I should play at Ramsden Park. They say that it's wonderful and have five courts set up for beginners, intermediate and advanced. That will be very interesting because in my winter pickleball we're all grouped together. Ramsden Park is about a half hour walk straight down the hill from my apartment, so I'm going! They have games during the day and in the evening. And the best part is that you don't need a partner; you just show up! But I'm sure that John will join me in the evenings. John will play tennis on the weekend, although I'm convinced that John will be a much better pickleballer than a tennis player and I think that he enjoys it more because there's a big social element to it.

Once a week I meet Donald and Sharon, my old friends from BMO, for lunch at Aroma.

A few times a week Pam and I go out for a walk and have some coffee after work hours because Pam is still working. And Pam and I see each other on the weekends and we go to the AGO and the ROM together.

On Thursday morning I walk to the grocery store with my grocery cart with wheels. I walk every Thursday (it's about a 20 minute walk each way) except for the days when we have snow so then I hop the streetcar.

On Fridays Sue and I have lunch at Daeco Sushi, but we've changed it to dinner because she educates children on how to play chess in French during the day. John now joins us for dinner and at times, so does Pam. We may change it back to lunch, depending on Sue's schedule.

On Saturdays Judy K. and I have lunch at the O&B Canteen on King St. It's a lovely place and they treat us like family.

Depending on what we're all doing I have dinner at Sue and John's on Saturday. We cook together, eat together and laugh together.

On either Saturday or Sunday afternoon Erik and I get together for coffee and a catch up.

I've learned to appreciate the world around me and I don't sweat the small stuff anymore! I used to really sweat the small stuff! Since I'm now living on pension I don't have much money to spend anymore, but it doesn't bother me. I still love to look around at fashion without feeling that I have to buy something. I'm not working anymore, so I don't need the wardrobe that I used to have. Sue and I love to go out on "fashion trips." And I still love makeup!

Before my stroke I only took a drug for my low thyroid. Now in addition to Levothyroxine for low thyroid, I am taking three drugs because of my stroke – Dabigatran is a blood thinner that I take twice a day, Diltiazem for heart rate control and Atorvastin for stroke prevention.

I really wanted to make sense of my stroke. I didn't want to just have a stroke and let it disappear. My stroke was a major part of my life and I wanted to do something to help people with what I've learned. I'm volunteering with the Aphasia Institute to help people that have had stokes because I really understand what they're going through! I've been there! **And I've written this book that will hopefully help people who've had a stroke. Or, if you have a friend or family member who's had a stroke, this book will hopefully help you too.**

Epilogue

As I'm lying on this magnificent beach in Mexico, I realized that my universe has made a full circle. Here I am, in perfect health, having a fabulous vacation with my friends; Willa – we were 13 when we met in Grade 8 homeroom, so we're now friends for 55 years! - and my best friend Sue. Who could ask for more?

My full circle started in 2017. Willa invited me to Marsh Harbor to go sailing. Marsh Harbor is a tiny island in the Bahamas and it's where she and her boyfriend kept their 43 foot sail boat. Willa has been living in Calgary for over 40 years and she loves getting away to warm climates in our Canadian winters. I was working at BMO at the time and I was delighted because I love anything to do with water and of course seeing Willa. I said, "YES!"

I flew down to Marsh Harbor where we had a fabulous holiday! We sailed and saw fabulous fish and manta rays. The weather was superb each and every day. I couldn't do much shopping because I travelled with a carry on, but I did find two very funky pairs of sunglasses. I'm addicted to sunglasses and I now have 29 pairs. I don't wear prescription glasses so I can afford this habit for which I don't pay more than $25.

Then came 2018 – my stroke! Then came COVID.

Now it's the end of 2022 and my friend Willa called. She and her boyfriend have rented a house for two months in Mexico, in the Yucatan Peninsula. Steve can only stay for six weeks and she has invited me to come to Mexico for the last 11 days. I tell Willa that I'm very sorry but I'm living on pension so I can't accept. Willa responds by telling me that she's taking care of my plane ticket, so I've got to say yes! And she told me that she wants to ask Sue to join us. Willa wanted to thank

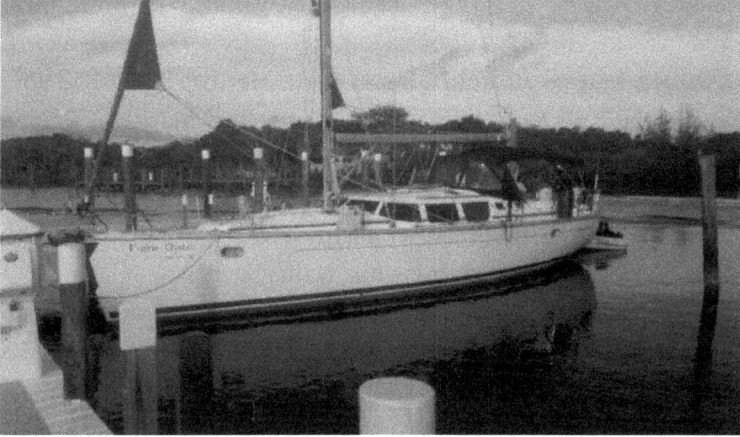

Here's a photo of the *Prairie Oyster* – their 43 foot sail boat.

Sue for everything that she did for me during my stroke and recovery. I was at Sue's while Willa and I were talking and Sue said, "YES!"

Sue and I are going to Mexico from February 6 -17, 2023. We've decided that we're travelling with a carry on only. And I've already booked a car service to the airport.

We have a flight that leaves for Merida at 6:30am, which mean that we have to be at the airport at 4:30am! The car service is picking us up at 3:30am.

We were flying to Merida and transiting through Dallas. Finally, we arrived in Merida, the capital of the Mexican state of Yucatan and the largest city in southeastern Mexico. Willa's house is in a small town approximately a 45 minute drive from Merida. There was Willa, greeting us! It was so exciting to finally see Willa for the first time in six years!

The house was beautiful! When you walked in there was a living room, dining room kitchen, two bathrooms and two bedrooms. Then there was sliding doors that opened onto a swimming pool and on the other side of the pool you walked into a living room, kitchen, bathroom and bedroom. Willa wanted the one bedroom part of the house in case she wakes up during the night and can't get back to sleep right away. So the three girls were all settled. The house was a two minute walk to the beach.

We decided that we should go and visit Merida. They had lots of museums, cathedrals, government buildings and markets. We went there on two separate days and had wonderful times.

Willa was getting a newsletter about things to do in the area. It said that we had to go to a town called Ticul. Everyone goes there to buy shoes. Can you imagine three girls not wanting to go to Ticul??? The interesting thing is that when you walk into a shoe store, they make their shoes in the back. So the only place you can buy these particular shoes is in this shoe store. And they only take pesos – no American dollars and no credit cards! We drove into Ticul and parked the car. In seconds a guy came over on a bike with a carriage in the front that could hold three people. He asked where we were going and we told him shoe shopping and he said that he'd take us. When we looked around, we saw a whole town full of these guys on bikes with carriages and with a license on the front. They were like taxis. We said, "Sure" and we headed off. He took us to fabulous shoe stores and the prices were unbelievable! Most of the shoes were between $10 and $20 Canadian dollars!!!

I bought beaded sandals for the equivalent of $22 Canadian dollars.

We then told our driver that we'd like to go for lunch, but not to a touristy place so he said that he'd take us to the place that he goes to eat. Naturally, we invited him to join us. It was absolutely WONDERFUL!!!!! And they had the best handmade fruit juices! The bill for the four of us was the equivalent of $30 Canadian dollars. Ticul was a **BIG HIT!!!**

We also went to Progreso, a larger town about 20 minutes from our house. Progreso was lovely, but it was full of tourists because the cruise liners stop there. The restaurants are more for tourists, but the food was very good.

We came to prefer the local restaurants near our house. They are completely open – no walls. There is a large, standing fan beside every table. If you're hot, you turn it on. And the food is fabulous and very

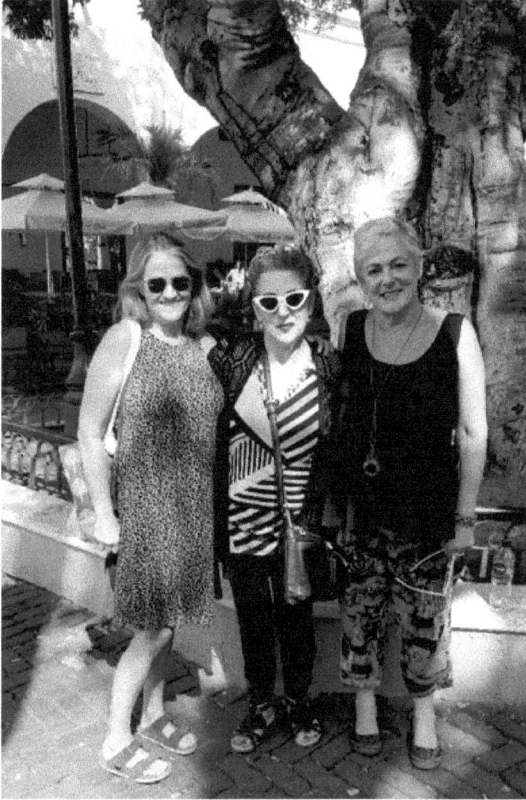

Sue, Me, and Willa in Merida.

cheap! I became addicted to coconut shrimp – about $20 Canadian dollars!

We had a wonderful 11 days and then it was time to say Adios to Mexico. This is a photo from our last night in Mexico. Of course I had coconut shrimp!

We all went to the airport together. When I went to say good-bye to Willa I started crying!! Sue and I went to catch our plane and after a miserable transit in Miami, we were home.

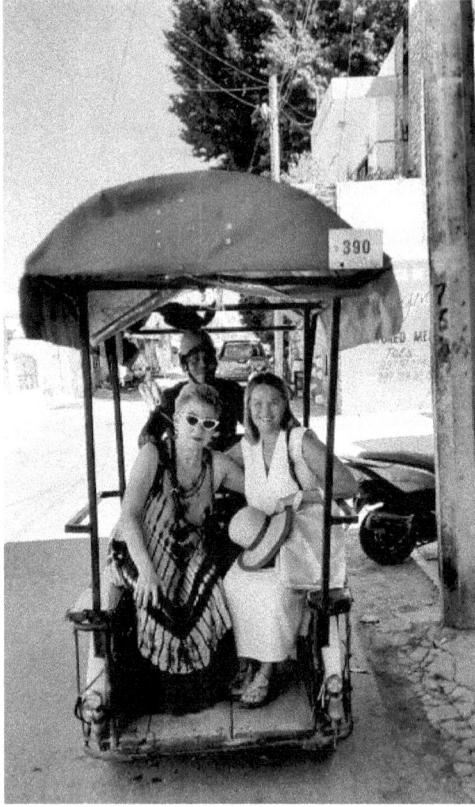

Here a photo of the guy who was our driver. That's Sue and
I sitting in the front waiting for Willa who bought eight pairs
of shoes.

Here's my circle - In 2017 when I went sailing with Willa, I was in
perfect health. And when I went to Mexico to be with Willa in 2023,
I was in perfect health. It's as if my stroke and recovery never happened.
But I will never forget my stroke and everything that I had to do to
recover! And I will never forget the help that I received from my friends
and of course most of all, everything that my best friend Sue did for
me, hence the title of the book – Two Friends & a Stroke!

Glossary of Terms

Stroke: A stroke happens when blood stops flowing to any part of your brain, damaging brain cells. The effects of a stroke depend on the part of the brain that was damaged and the amount of damage done.

Ischemic strokes: These are strokes caused by blockage of an artery (or, in rare instances, a vein). About 87% of all strokes are ischemic.

Hemorrhagic strokes: These are strokes caused by bleeding. About 13% of all strokes are hemorrhagic.

Silent stroke: It's a stroke without any noticeable symptoms.

Aphasia: It's a condition that robs you of your ability to communicate – speak, write and understand language, both verbal and written.

Atrial Fibrillation or AFib: It's an irregular heartbeat (quiver) in the atria which could prevent all of the blood flowing down to the ventricle – could cause blood clots.

Anticoagulant: Blood thinner.

Dabigatran: Anticoagulant used to treat and prevent blood clots and to prevent strokes in people with AFib.

Diltiazem: It's a channel blocker that works by relaxing the muscles of your heart and blood vessels. It's used to treat certain heart rhythm disorders.

Atorvastin: It belongs to a certain group of medicines called statins. It's taken to prevent heart attacks and strokes.

Tissue plasminogen activator (tPA): It's the main treatment for an ischemic stroke. It breaks up the blood clots that block blood flow to your brain. A doctor will inject tPA into a vein in your arm. This type of medicine must be given within 3 hours after your symptoms start.

Neuroplasticity: Neuroplasticity is the brain's ability to change and adapt due to experience. It is an umbrella term referring to the brain's ability to change, reorganize, or grow neural networks. This can involve functional changes due to brain damage or structural changes due to learning.

Plasticity refers to the brain's malleability or ability to change; it does not imply that the brain is plastic. *Neuro* refers to neurons, the nerve cells that are the building blocks of the brain and nervous system. Thus, neuroplasticity allows nerve cells to change or adjust.

Acknowledgments

There are so many people that I'd like to thank! I couldn't have recovered without all of you!

My beloved parents Shirley and Joe. Throughout my whole life, I was SO loved! Shirley stayed alive and saved me when I had my stroke. Joe taught me how to live my life happily, no matter what was going on. He used to wake up every day, smile and say, "Thank you. I've made another day." I do the same. THANK YOU!

My best friend Sue Foster. I really had no idea what a best friend was until I had my stroke. You were always there for me, every minute of every day. I never had to ask, but you always knew what I needed and you made sure that I had it. I could never have recovered, if not for you. That's why this book is called *Two Friends*. We did everything together! THANK YOU!

My closest friends in Toronto – Pam, Katherine and Everton, Judy K., and Sonya - that did so much for me while I was recovering. I am forever in your debt! THANK YOU!

My two favourite doctors - Dr. Daniel Selchen of St. Michael's Hospital and Dr. Heather MacNeill of Bridgepoint Rehab. They gave me such outstanding care! THANK YOU!

My speech therapist, my occupational therapist and my physiotherapist – inpatient and outpatient – at Bridgepoint. Thanks to you, I learned how to speak again, walk again and got back the full use of my right arm and hand. I will never forget everything that you did for me! THANK YOU!

My yoga friends - Ronit and Daniel Wilk of Oxygen Yoga & Fitness and their fabulous instructors. When I wanted to start yoga one year after I had my stroke, I had no sense of balance and my right arm and hand were very weak. Ronit told me that yoga is for everyone, just tell the instructors before you start the class. The instructors were FABULOUS and I still go six times a week. THANK YOU!

My dear friend Gregory Cheadle. He encouraged, supported and guided me for my book. And, he steered me in the direction of my Agent, Alan Morell. THANK YOU!

My uberAgent, Alan Morell of THE CREATIVE MANAGEMENT AGENCY in Beverly Hills, CA. Alan believed in me and sold my book to a prestigious Publisher. THANK YOU!

My Publisher, John T. Colby, Brick Tower Press. John shared my vision for wanting to get my story out that love, friends and family give you hope and inspiration to win back your life. THANK YOU!

For sales, editorial information, subsidiary rights information
or a catalog, please write or phone or e-mail
Brick Tower Press
Manhanset House
Shelter Island Hts., New York 11965, US
Tel: 212-427-7139
www.BrickTowerPress.com
bricktower@aol.com
www.IngramContent.com

For sales in the UK and Europe please contact our distributor,
Gazelle Book Services
White Cross Mills
Lancaster, LA1 4XS, UK
Tel: (01524) 68765 Fax: (01524) 63232
email: jacky@gazellebooks.co.uk

www.ingramcontent.com/pod-product-compliance
Lightning Source LLC
Chambersburg PA
CBHW071951260326
41914CB00004B/785

* 9 7 8 1 8 7 6 9 6 9 1 0 3 *